Understand Your Diabetes...
and Live a Healthy Life

Understand Your Diabetes...
and Live a Healthy Life

Diabetes Day-Care Unit, Hôtel-Dieu Hospital, Montreal

In collaboration with Dr. Robert G. Josse
Division of Endocrinology and Metabolism, St. Michael's Hospital
Professor of Medicine, University of Toronto

Second edition
Revised and expanded

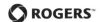 **ROGERS**™

Library and Archives Canada Cataloguing in Publication
Main entry under title:
   Understand your diabetes ... and live a healthy life
   2nd ed. Rev. and augm.
   Translation of: Connaître son diabète... pour mieux vivre
   ISBN: 2-922260-16-X

   1. Diabetes – Popular works. 2. Diabetics – health and hygiene.
   3. Diabetes – Diet therapy. 4. Diabete – Prevention. I. Chiasson,
   Jean-Louis. II. CHUM. Hôtel-Dieu. Unité de jour de diabète.

   RC660.4.C6613 2004   616.4'62   C2004- 941792-4

Translation: Mark Lepage

English editing : Brent Woodford and Geneviève Roquet

Graphic design: Folio infographie

Layout: Lucie Benoit

Cover design: Dino Peressini

© Diabetes Day-Care Unit, Hôtel-Dieu Hospital, CHUM, 2001

© Rogers Media, 2004
1200 McGill College avenue, suite 800
Montreal, Quebec H3B 4G7
Tel.: (514) 845-5141 / Fax : (514) 843-2183

Legal Deposit: 3rd quarter 2004
Bibliothèque nationale du Québec, 2004
National Library of Canada, 2004

The publication of this work was made possible thanks to an unrestricted
educational grant from Aventis Pharma.

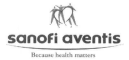

Foreword

The time has come for the second edition of *Understand Your Diabetes... and Live a Healthy Life*. Our understanding of the disease, its causes, its diagnosis, its complications, its treatment and especially its prevention is rapidly evolving. It is important that both people with diabetes and those at risk of developing the disease remain well informed. On the one hand, people at risk must be motivated to change their lifestyle in order to prevent the appearance of the disease; on the other hand, it is important to help people with diabetes take responsibility for their treatment and achieve optimal control of their blood glucose in order to prevent complications in both the short and long terms.

This second edition features a great deal of new information for the general population as well as for people with diabetes. For the first time, we outline the risk factors implicated in the development of diabetes and discuss the prevention of type 2 diabetes. For people with diabetes, we have provided an update of the latest blood glucose meters available for purchase, indicating which ones allow blood samples to be taken from sites other than the fingertip. We have also included an update on oral antidiabetic medications and insulins. As for nutrition, we offer the new nutritional guidelines released by Health Canada. The treatment of diabetes requires that the patient be proactive, and modify his or her lifestyle accordingly. This requires a lot of motivation, and we have therefore included a chapter on that subject.

We hope that this book will be a source of information for the general population and that it will motivate people suffering from diabetes to take charge of their health, to understand themselves better, to improve their treatment and to live healthy lives.

The team of the Diabetes Day-Care Unit, Hôtel-Dieu Hospital, Montreal

From the same publisher*

Dr. Michael McCormack and Dr. Fred Saad
Understanding Prostate Cancer (2004)

Dr. André-H. Dandavino *et al.*
The Family Guide to Symptoms, 2nd edition (2003)

Dr. Michael McCormack *et al.*
Male Sexual Health (2003)

Dr. André-H. Dandavino *et al.*
The Family Guide to Health Problems (2001)

Dr. Jacques Boulay
Bilingual Guide to Medical Abbreviations, 3rd edition (1998)

* All the above titles are also available in French.

Authors

This work was re-edited by members of the Diabetes Day-Care Unit Multidisciplinary team at Hôtel-Dieu Hospital, Montreal:

Jean-Louis Chiasson, endocrinologist
Françoise Desrochers, registered nurse
Lyne Gauthier, pharmacist
Nicole Hamel, pharmacist
Michelle Messier, dietician
Charles Tourigny, psychologist

We would also like to acknowledge the contributions of the authors of previous editions:

Nathalie Beaulieu, dietician
Julie Demers, pharmacist
Micheline Fecteau-Côté, dietician
Sylvie Fournier, pharmacist
Christiane Gobeil, dietician
Lise Lussier, psychologist
Caroline Rivest, pharmacist
Danièle Tremblay, psychologist
Francis Viguié, psychologist

Acknowledgments

We would like to extend our heartfelt thanks to members of the Endocrinology, Metabolism and Nutrition divisions of Hôtel-Dieu Hospital for their contributions. We also thank Catherine Noulard and Thérèse Surprenant of Hôtel-Dieu Hospital for their savvy of editing the dietetic content of this book, and Susanne Bordeleau for her inspirational work organizing and coordinating this effort. Moreover, we would like to thank Marie-Claire Barbeau, Geneviève Côté and Louise Tremblay of Diabetes Québec for their insightful editing as well as their helpful comments and suggestions concerning the text.

Objectives of This Book

The objectives of this book are as follows:

General objective

To enable people with diabetes to acquire optimal control of their health in order to limit the time they spend in the hospital and to lower their chances of developing complications related to diabetes.

Specific objectives

To enable people with diabetes to adopt lifestyle habits which facilitate the maintenance of normal blood glucose levels, and to help them to:

1) acquire general knowledge about diabetes;

2) adapt their diet according to their diabetes and their activities;

3) take into account the effects of stress and exercise on the control of their illness;

4) recognize the complications that are caused by poor blood glucose control;

5) take action if and when these complications do arise;

6) take medications as prescribed;

7) understand the importance of foot care and to adopt general hygiene measures;

8) utilize devices for measuring blood glucose levels;

9) use community resources as needed;

10) develop a positive attitude when taking charge of their condition.

Contents

CHAPTER 1

General Information on Diabetes

1. What is diabetes?

Diabetes is a disease characterized by **an elevation of blood glucose level** (or blood sugar level) above normal.

2. How many Canadians are affected by diabetes?

About **two million Canadians** (7% of the population) have diabetes, but close to half of them remain undiagnosed and unaware of their condition. It is anticipated that the number of cases will have doubled by 2025, making diabetes **the disease of the twenty-first century** and generating increasingly significant costs, currently estimated at close to $9 billion per year in Canada. Diabetes is a growing societal problem that must be battled on all fronts.

3. What are the criteria for diagnosing diabetes?

The diagnosis of diabetes is based on results of the following lab tests conducted on venous blood:

1) **fasting blood glucose** equal to or above 7.0 mmol/l;

2) **random blood glucose** equal to or above 11.1 mmol/l;

3)   **oral glucose tolerance test,** with a blood glucose level equal to or above 11.1 mmol/l two hours after the consumption of 75 g of glucose.

However, a doctor's diagnosis of diabetes requires that an abnormal value from one of these tests be confirmed on a different day by repeating any one of these tests.

4.   What is normal blood glucose?

Blood glucose is considered normal when it remains steady **between 4 mmol/l and 6 mmol/l before meals and between 5 mmol/l and 8 mmol/l one to two hours after meals.**

5.   What are the blood glucose levels targeted in the treatment of diabetes?

The majority of people with diabetes should aim for a **target glucose level** between 4 mmol/l and 7 mmol/l before meals and between 5 mmol/l and 10 mmol/l one or two hours after meals. However, in cases where there is no risk, a person with diabetes should aim **for a normal glucose level** between 4 mmol/l and 6 mmol/l before meals and between 5 mmol/l and 8 mmol/l one or two hours after meals.

6.   Why is it important to achieve a normal or target blood glucose level?

The closer blood glucose is to normal, the more a person with diabetes will:

1)   feel fit, and

2)   lower the risks of long-term complications associated with diabetes.

7.   Why do blood glucose levels increase in a person with diabetes?

Blood glucose rises because of a **lack of insulin action, which may be due to reduced insulin production**. In such cases, there is not enough insulin to allow glucose to enter the cells, and the level of glucose in the blood increases as a result. This is called **hyperglycemia**.

8. What is insulin?

Insulin is a hormone produced by the **pancreas**, an organ located in the abdomen, behind the stomach.

One might say that insulin is the **key that opens the door and allows glucose to enter the cells,** and this helps to lower the blood glucose.

9. What is glucose used for in the body?

Glucose is an important **energy source** for the body's cells, in the same way that gasoline is the prime energy source for cars.

10. What is the source of excess glucose in the blood of a person with diabetes?

Excess glucose in the blood comes from two main sources:

1) **foods containing carbohydrates** consumed during meals and snacks;

2) the **liver**, which stores glucose at mealtime and releases it into the blood between meals.

11. What are the characteristics of type 1 diabetes?

Type 1 diabetes is usually characterized by the following features:

1) **total absence of insulin**;

2) appearance of the disease **toward the onset of puberty** and usually **before the age 40**;

3) **weight loss**;

4) the need for treatment with **insulin injections**.

12. What are the characteristics of type 2 diabetes?

Type 2 diabetes is generally characterized by the following features:

1) **insulin resistance**, when the insulin produced becomes less effective;

2) insufficiency of insulin production to compensate for the insulin's reduced effectiveness;

3) appearance of the disease after the age of 40;

4) **excess weight**;

5) the need for a **dietary program, alone** or combined with **oral antidiabetic medication; insulin injections** may become necessary.

13. Are some people predisposed to diabetes?

Yes. Susceptibility to diabetes is inherited genetically.

14. Are there factors that may trigger diabetes in those predisposed to the disease?

Yes, a number of factors may trigger the disease in those predisposed to it. In type 1 diabetes, factors such as a viral infection may precipitate the disease in a susceptible person. In type 2 diabetes, two major factors can play important roles in the development of the disease: excess weight and lack of physical activity. Physical or physiological stresses may also cause predisposed individuals to develop diabetes, especially type 2; these include heart attacks, a cerebrovascular accidents (strokes) or infections. Psychological stress, for instance the loss of a loved one, may also bring on the disease. Certain medications, for instance high doses of cortisone, can also act as triggers.

15. Can some diseases cause diabetes?

Yes, certain diseases may cause diabetes. Cystic fibrosis and pancreatitis (inflammation of the pancreas) may destroy the pancreas and bring on diabetes. Other conditions, such as gestational diabetes, polycystic ovary syndrome and certain types of muscular dystrophy, as well as some endocrine diseases such as Cushing's disease or acromegaly, also increase the risk of developing diabetes.

16. Are there tests to identify people who are predisposed to develop type 2 diabetes?

There are tests that identify people with an elevated risk of developing the disease.

A fasting blood glucose level above 6 mmol/l but below 7 mmol/l is considered an **abnormal fasting blood glucose level**, called **impaired fasting blood glucose**. Also, an oral glucose tolerance test, which consists of drinking a beverage containing 75 g of glucose on an empty stomach, may indicate glucose intolerance if blood glucose measures between 7.8 mmol/l and 11.0 mmol/l two hours after the test.

These two conditions, **impaired fasting blood glucose** and **impaired glucose tolerance**, are considered "pre-diabetic" and indicate an elevated risk of developing the disease.

17. Is it possible to prevent or slow down the development of diabetes in pre-diabetic people?

Yes, it has been demonstrated that in people who have present glucose intolerance, weight loss and physical activity may decrease the risk of developing type 2 diabetes by over 50%. Certain medications (metformine and acarbose) have also been shown to be effective, decreasing the risk of developing diabetes in subjects with impaired glucose tolerance by over 30%.

18. How can a person with diabetes reach and maintain a target or normal blood glucose level?

To control diabetes, the person dealing with the disease must take responsibility for his or her own treatment. The following guidelines may prove useful in this regard:

1)   acknowledge and accept the condition;

2)   eat healthy food;

3)   follow a mild weight loss program, if necessary;

4)   follow a regular physical activity regimen;

5)   regularly measure **blood glucose**;

6)   take antidiabetic **medications** as prescribed;

7)   learn to **manage** stress;

8)   stay **well informed** about diabetes.

➡ The person best able to control your diabetes is you—with the help and support of your doctor and other health care professionals.

➡ Diabetes is a chronic disease: it cannot be cured, but it can be controlled.

➡ You have done nothing to bring on your diabetes; you have nothing to feel guilty about.

➡ The closer you keep your blood glucose to normal, the better you will feel.

➡ Finding out about diabetes allows you to take more responsibility for your condition.

CHAPTER 2

Hyperglycemia

1. What is hyperglycemia?

Hyperglycemia occurs when the blood glucose rises above target levels, that is, above 7mmol/L before meals and 10 mmol/l one or two hours after meals.

2. How do people with diabetes develop hyperglycemia?

People with diabetes develop hyperglycemia when **the amount of insulin in the blood is not sufficient to handle the amount of glucose being released into the bloodstream.**

3. What are the symptoms of hyperglycemia?

When blood glucose rises above a certain threshold, the following symptoms may appear:

1) **increase in the volume of urine and the frequency of urination**;

2) intense **thirst**;

3) dry **mouth**;

4) excessive **hunger**;

5) involuntary **weight loss**.

Hyperglycemia may also lead to the following symptoms:

6) blurred vision;

7) infections, especially of the genital organs and bladder;

8) wounds that do not heal well;

9) fatigue;

10) sleepiness;

11) irritability.

4.   What are the main causes of hyperglycemia?

The primary causes of hyperglycemia are:

1) excessive consumption of **foods containing carbohydrates;**

2) a decrease in physical activity;

3) incorrect dosage of antidiabetic medications (insulin or pills);

4) an infection;

5) poor **stress** management;

6) taking certain **medications** like cortisone;

7) uncorrected **nocturnal hypoglycemia (low blood sugar)** followed by a hyperglycemic rebound in the morning (see chapter 18).

5.   What must a person with diabetes do when hyperglycemia is suspected?

When a person with diabetes suspects hyperglycemia, it is important that he or she do the following:

1) measure blood glucose;

2) people with type 1 diabetes must **check for the presence of ketone bodies** if blood glucose is higher than 14 mmol/l. Use Ketostix® reagent strips to measure the level of ketone bodies in urine, and the Precision Xtra™ meter by MediSense® to measure the level of ketone bodies in a blood sample taken from the fingertip;

3) **drink plenty of water** to avoid dehydration (250 ml of water per hour, unless contraindicated);

4) identify the cause of the hyperglycemia;

5) correct the cause if possible;

6) continue eating (including carbohydrates) and follow the prescribed treatment (antidiabetic oral medications or insulin);

7) call the doctor or go to the emergency department if:

➤ blood glucose rises above 20 mmol/l; or

➤ the presence of ketone bodies in the urine average (4 mmol/l) to high (16 mmo/L); or

➤ the presence of ketone bodies in a blood sample taken from the fingertip is above 3 mmol/l; or

➤ it is impossible to retain liquids taken orally because of nausea and vomiting.

6. What are the long-term complications associated with hyperglycemia?

In the long term, hyperglycemia may lead to complications affecting the eyes, kidneys, nerves, heart and blood vessels.

CHAPTER 3

Hypoglycemia and Glucagon

1. What is hypoglycemia?

Hypoglycemia is a drop in blood glucose levels **below normal**, or below 4 mmol/l.

2. Why does a person with diabetes develop hypoglycemia?

A person with diabetes develops hypoglycemia when, as a result of treatment, **there is too much insulin in the blood relative to the amount of glucose entering the circulation.**

3. Who is susceptible to hypoglycemia?

People **who inject insulin or who take medications that stimulate the pancreas to produce more insulin**, such as chlorpropamide (Apo®-Chlorpropamide), tolbutamide (Apo^MD-Tolbutamide), glyburide (Diabeta®, Euglucon®), gliclazide (Diamicron® and Diamicron® MR), glimepiride (Amaryl®), repaglinide (GlucoNorm®) and nateglinide (Starlix®), may develop hypoglycemia.

4.   What are the symptoms of hypoglycemia?

Our body has two types of warning systems. The first one results in symptoms that occur **rapidly**, brought on by the secretion of adrenalin.

When hypoglycemia occurs rapidly, it may produce the following symptoms:

1)   **tremors or shakes;**

2)   **palpitations;**

3)   **sweating or perspiration;**

4)   **anxiety;**

5)   **acute hunger;**

6)   **paleness;**

7)   **nightmares and restless sleep**, if the hypoglycemia occurs during sleep;

8)   **waking with a headache** and rebound **hyperglycemia** in the morning following uncorrected nocturnal hypoglycemia (during the previous night's sleep).

The second warning system results in less perceptible symptoms that develop more **slowly**. These symptoms are due to a lack of glucose in the brain.

When hypoglycemia occurs **slowly**, the symptoms are more subtle:

1)   **numbness or tingling around the mouth;**

2)   **yawning;**

3)   **fatigue or weakness;**

4)   **the urge to sleep;**

5)   **mood swings;**

6)   **aggressiveness;**

7)   **dizziness;**

8) blurred vision;

9) unsteady gait, poor coordination;

10) difficulty pronouncing words;

11) confusion.

5. Does hypoglycemia necessarily result in all these symptoms?

No. The symptoms of hypoglycemia vary from one person to another and may change over time. Sometimes, a person with diabetes may develop hypoglycemia without symptoms, especially if the blood glucose level decreases slowly, or the diabetes has existed for many years, and hypoglycemia is no longer effectively appreciated.

6. What causes hypoglycemia?

The most frequent causes of hypoglycemia, sorted into four categories, are:

1) food

➤ skipping a snack or a meal;

➤ delaying a meal;

➤ lower-than-required consumption of foods containing carbohydrates;

➤ an error in measuring the level of carbohydrates in food;

➤ inability to keep food down (vomiting, diarrhea);

➤ consuming alcohol, which may cause hypoglycemia as long as 16 hours after its consumption;

➤ fasting when taking antidiabetic medications;

➤ gastroparesis (delayed emptying of the content of the stomach);

2)   **physical activity**

➤   physical activity without adjusting food or medication intake;

3)   **stress**

➤   an excessive increase in physical activity (e.g., a long walk, brisk house cleaning) in an attempt to manage stress;

4)   **antidiabetic medications**

➤   incorrect (excessive) dosage of antidiabetic medications or insulin;

➤   overcorrecting elevated blood glucose by injecting an excessive dose of insulin;

➤   failing to adjust to a lower dosage despite blood glucose levels frequently lower than 4 mmol/l;

➤   taking antidiabetic medications at the wrong time.

7.   What should the person with diabetes do when hypoglycemia is suspected?

When a person with diabetes suspects the onset of hypoglycemia, he or she should never assume that the blood glucose level will correct itself. The person with diabetes **must not go to sleep. Rather, he or she must:**

1)   **measure the blood glucose level;**

2)   **eat food that supplies 15 g of carbohydrates** and can be absorbed rapidly. Glucose or sucrose, in pill or liquid form, is preferable;

3)   **avoid overtreating the hypoglycemia:**

➤   **wait 15 minutes;**

➤   **measure the blood glucose again** and, if the hypoglycemia persists, **consume an additional 15 g of carbohydrates;**

If the hypoglycemia is corrected but the next meal is more than an hour away, add a snack containing 15 g of carbohydrates and a protein source (e.g., 300 ml of milk or 7 soda crackers with cheese, or fruit with cheese).

4)   If the person with diabetes **is unable to administer his or her own treatment**:

➤   if possible, measure the blood glucose level;

➤   give him or her some food supplying **20 g of carbohydrates**;

➤   repeat as needed after 15 minutes with food containing 15 g of carbohydrates if blood glucose remains lower than 4 mmol/l.

Examples of foods supplying 15 g of carbohydrates:

1st choice (absorbed quickly)

➤   3 tablets of Glucose BD ® (1 tablet = 5 g of carbohydrates)

➤   5 tablets of Dextrosol® (1 tablet = 3 g of carbohydrates)

➤   7 tablets of Glucosol™ (1 tablet = 2.25 g of carbohydrates)

➤   125 ml ($^1/_2$ cup) of regular soft drink (not diet) or fruit beverage

➤   5 ml (3 teaspoons or 3 packets) of sugar dissolved in water

➤   15 ml (3 teaspoons) of honey, jam or syrup

2nd choice (absorbed more slowly)

➤   125 ml ($^1/_2$ cup) of fruit juice without added sugar

➤   300 ml ($1^1/_4$ cups) of milk

➤   200 ml (1 single-serving size carton) of milk with 2 "Social Tea" biscuits

➤   4 "Social Tea" biscuits

➤   7 soda crackers

➤   1 dried fruit bar (e.g., "Fruit To Go")

➤   1 small apple, $^1/_2$ banana, 2 kiwis or 2 dates, etc.

Examples of foods containing **20 g of carbohydrates** that are absorbed more quickly:

➡ 4 tablets of Glucose BD® (1 tablet = 5 g of carbohydrates)

➡ 7 tablets of Dextrosol® (1 tablet = 3 g of carbohydrates)

➡ 9 tablets of Glucosol™ (1 tablet = 2.25 g of carbohydrates)

➡ 20 ml (4 teaspoons) of honey, jam or syrup

➡ 20 ml (4 teaspoons) or 4 packets of sugar dissolved in water

➡ 175 ml (³/₄ cup) of regular soft drink (not diet) or fruit beverage

8.   Why is it important to treat hypoglycemia immediately?

It is very important to treat any episode of hypoglycemia **immediately**, because if left uncorrected hypoglycemia may lead to loss of consciousness, coma and sometimes even convulsions. Hypoglycemia, no matter how severe it is, must always be taken seriously.

9.   Does uncorrected hypoglycemia necessarily lead to coma?

No, uncorrected hypoglycemia does not necessarily lead to coma. During hypoglycemia, the body will attempt to defend itself by secreting hormones such as glucagon and adrenalin. These hormones may elevate blood glucose and correct hypoglycemia. However, if there is too much insulin in the blood, these defensive reflexes may not be sufficient to correct the hypoglycemia and prevent a coma.

10. How can hypoglycemia be avoided?

Hypoglycemia can generally be avoided by taking the following precautions:

1)   measure blood glucose regularly;

2)   keep regular mealtime hours and include foods containing carbohydrates;

3)   check blood glucose before undertaking any physical activity and consume carbohydrates as necessary (see chapter 20 on physical activity);

4)   avoid consuming alcohol on an empty stomach;

5)   check blood glucose around 2 a.m., as necessary;

6)   take antidiabetic medications as prescribed, respecting the recommended dosage and timetable;

7)   people with type 1 diabetes are advised to periodically check blood glucose around 2 a.m. A bedtime snack containing at least 15 g of carbohydrates and a protein source is also recommended before turning in for the night, if blood glucose is below 7 mmol/l at that time.

11. What safety measures must be taken by a person with diabetes at risk for hypoglycemia?

The person with diabetes at risk for hypoglycemia must:

1)   always have at least two **15 g servings of carbohydrates** handy;

2)   wear a **bracelet or a pendant** identifying him or her as diabetic;

3)   **forewarn** family, friends and work colleagues that he or she has diabetes. Inform them of the symptoms of hypoglycemia and the means to remedy it;

4)   always have **glucagon** on hand at home, at work or when travelling if he or she takes insulin. A friend or relative must learn how to inject the glucagon should the person with diabetes fall into a hypoglycemic coma.

12. What must be done if a person with diabetes is in a hypoglycemic coma?

If a person with diabetes is unconscious or in a hypoglycemic coma, you must:

1)   inject him or her with glucagon, if available; if not,

2)   call an ambulance.

Never attempt to feed sugary foods to an unconscious person. Food may go into the lungs instead of the stomach.

13. What is glucagon?

Glucagon is a hormone produced by the pancreas to elevate blood glucose. In the event of a hypoglycemic coma, glucagon must be injected by another person in order to correct the hypoglycemia.

Have a "glucagon injection" first-aid kit on hand, which can be stored at room temperature. Check the expiry date periodically.

Here are the steps to folllow in the event of a hypoglycemic coma:

1) lay an unconscious diabetic person on his or her side, as glucagon may cause nausea and vomiting;

2) remove the plastic cap from the bottle of glucagon;

3) remove the needle sheath and inject the entire contents of the syringe into the bottle of glucagon. Do not remove the plastic stop ring from the syringe. Remove the syringe from the bottle;

4) gently shake the bottle until the glucagon powder is completely dissolved in the solvent;

5) draw up all of the solution from the vial using the same syringe;

6) inject the contents of the syringe (1 mg) subcutaneously (under the skin) or intramuscularly. The person should awaken within 15 minutes. There is no risk of overdose. A doctor may recommend a half dose for children under five;

7) feed the person with diabetes as soon as he or she is awake and able to swallow. Provide a substantial snack containing 45 g of carbohydrates and a source of protein, such as a fast sugar (e.g., a soft drink or fruit beverage) **and** a slow sugar (e.g., crackers and cheese or a meat sandwich);

8) advise the diabetic person's doctor of the incident so that treatment can be evaluated and possibly adjusted.

> If the person with diabetes does not regain consciousness within 15 to 20 minutes after the glucagon injection, see that he or she is transported to the emergency department immediately.

14. What advice can be offered to a person with diabetes who lives alone and is at risk for nocturnal hypoglycemia?

A person with diabetes living alone may have considerable fear of nocturnal hypoglycemia. However, hypoglycemia rarely persists for extended periods of time. In a crisis situation, the body reacts by raising the blood glucose level, using sugar stored in the liver. Nevertheless, the situation is stressful. Therefore, in addition to taking preventative measures to avoid crises, a person with diabetes should also develop a help network to ensure his or her safety in case of prolonged hypoglycemia. Here are some suggestions:

1) ask a friend or relative to phone every morning;

2) ask the mailman to deliver the mail in person;

3) agree on a code system with a neighbour (e.g., one curtain open or closed upon waking);

4) use a personal response telephone service with a two-way voice communication system such as Argus Lifeline: (514) 735-2101 or 1 888 517-3387.

> It is wise to leave a house key with a friend or relative who can provide assistance as needed.

15. Can symptoms of hypoglycemia occur when blood glucose is normal?

Yes, a person with diabetes can have symptoms of hypoglycemia when blood glucose is normal, in these two situations:

1) When hyperglycemia has existed for some time, using antidiabetic medications to normalize blood glucose levels may trigger symptoms of hypoglycemia lasting several days (especially if the blood sugar falls from high to normal too quickly). In order to avoid this unpleasant situation, it may be necessary to allow the blood glucose level to rise and then to lower it gradually. Nonetheless, it is important to regain a normal blood glucose level.

2) When the blood glucose level is very elevated and then drops rapidly to normal, a person may experience symptoms of hypoglycemia that fade quickly. It is therefore important to always test blood glucose levels when hypoglycemia is suspected, in order to avoid treating a false case of hypoglycemia and thus triggering hyperglycemia.

16. Is reactive hypoglycemia a sign of diabetes?

Reactive hypoglycemia sometimes occurs as the first sign of type 2 diabetes. This type of hypoglycemia usually appears three or four hours after a meal containing carbohydrates – hence the term "reactive". In general, reactive hypoglycemia corrects itself spontaneously, even if no carbohydrates are ingested.

➤ The symptoms or signs of hypoglycemia do not always occur together at the same time.

➤ The symptoms of hypoglycemia differ from one person to the next.

➤ Symptoms and discomforts may change over time. When a person has been diabetic for 10 to 20 years, he or she may no longer experience the symptoms of hypoglycemia (neuropathy).

➤ The symptoms of hypoglycemia may be masked if the diabetic person takes certain medications, such as beta-blockers.

➤ The symptoms of hypoglycemia may be absent in the case of repeated episodes.

➤ Certain signs and symptoms of hypoglycemia are difficult to evaluate. It is therefore preferable to confirm glucose levels with a glucose meter in order to avoid making an unnecessary correction.

➤ It is recommended that hypoglycemia be corrected immediately, by following the prescribed steps, in order to ensure that there is no damage to the brain. Remember, that hypoglycemia, no matter how severe it is, must always be taken seriously.

Recommendations for the treatment of hypoglycemia for people with diabetes

Test the blood glucose level immediately

↓

If the blood glucose level is below 4.0 mmol/l

↓

1. **If no assistance is required for treatment,
    take 15 g of carbohydrates, in the appropriate from:**

1st choice (absorbed quickly)

- ➤ 3 tablets of Glucose BD® (1 tablet = 5 g of carbohydrates)

- ➤ 5 tablets of Dextrosol® (1 tablet = 3 g of carbohydrates)

- ➤ 7 tablets of Glucosol™ (1 tablet = 2.25 g of carbohydrates)

- ➤ 125 ml (¹/₂ cup) of regular soft drink or fruit beverage

- ➤ 15 ml (3 teaspoons or 3 packets) of sugar dissolved in water

- ➤ 15 ml (3 teaspoons) of honey, jam or syrup

2nd choice (absorbed more slowly)

- ➤ 125 ml (¹/₂ cup) of fruit juice without added sugar

- ➤ 300 ml (1¹/₄ cups) of milk

- ➤ 200 ml (1 single-serving-size carton) of milk, plus 2 "Social Tea" biscuits

- ➤ 4 "Social Tea" biscuits

- ➤ 7 soda crackers

- ➤ 1 dried fruit bar (e.g., "Fruit To Go")

- ➤ 1 small apple, ¹/₂ banana, 2 kiwis or 2 dates, etc.

2. **If the person is conscious but assistance is required for treatment, give 20 g of carbohydrates in the appropriate form:**

➤ 4 tablets of Glucose BD® (1 tablet = 5 g of carbohydrates)

➤ 7 tablets of Dextrosol® (1 tablet = 3 g of carbohydrates)

➤ 9 tablets of Glucosol™ (1 tablet = 2.25 g of carbohydrates)

➤ 20 ml (4 teaspoons) of honey, jam or syrup

➤ 20 ml (4 teaspoons or 4 packets) of sugar dissolved in water

➤ 175 ml (³/₄ cup) of regular soft drink or fruit beverage

↓

Wait 15 minutes and test the blood glucose level again

↓

If the blood glucose level is still below 4.0 mmol/l,

take another 15 g of carbohydrates

↓

Wait 15 minutes and repeat the treatment as needed

↓

When the blood glucose level reaches or exceeds 4.0 mmol/l

↓

Meal (or snack) expected within an hour or less

↓   ↓

Yes, have the meal or snack as planned.	**No,** have a snack containing 15 g of carbohydrates and a protein source (e.g., 200 ml of milk, plus 2 "Social Tea" biscuits) while waiting for the meal.

3.   If the person with diabetes is unconscious:

➤ Inject 1 mg of Glucagon SC or IM (dosage for adults and children over five).

➤ When the person with diabetes has regained consciousness and can swallow, provide a substantial snack of 45 g of carbohydrates and a protein source (e.g., orange juice and a meat sandwich).

Caution

1.   For people with diabetes taking acarbose (Prandase®) in combination with other medications that may cause hypoglycemia, it is recommended that hypoglycemia be corrected in one of the following ways:

➤ 3 tablets of Glucose BD® (1 tablet = 5 g of carbohydrates), or

➤ 5 tablets of Dextrosol® (1 tablet = 3 g of carbohydrates)

➤ 300 ml (1¼ cups) of milk, or

➤ 15 ml (3 teaspoons) of honey

2.   For people with diabetes suffering from kidney problems, it is recommended that hypoglycemia be corrected in one of the following ways:

➤ 3 tablets of Glucose BD® (1 tablet = 5 g of carbohydrates)

➤ 5 tablets of Dextrosol® (1 tablet = 3 g of carbohydrates)

➤ 3 packets of sugar dissolved in a little water

3.   Hypoglycemia should never be dismissed as slight or unimportant. All appropriate measures should be taken to prevent it, and when it occurs, it must be treated immediately.

CHAPTER 4

Self-Monitoring: Blood Glucose and Glycosylated Hemoglobin

1. What is self-monitoring?

Self-monitoring is a technique used by the person with diabetes to **measure his or her own blood glucose level**. Generally, the approach also includes adjusting the treatment according to the results thus obtained, in order to bring and maintain the blood glucose level as close to normal as possible.

2. Why use self-monitoring?

Self-monitoring allows a person with diabetes to:

1)   check the impact of **nutrition, physical activity, stress and antidiabetic medications** on blood glucose;

2)   identify episodes of hypoglycemia and hyperglycemia, and take rapid action;

3) modify his or her behaviour with respect to nutrition, physical activity, antidiabetic medications and stress, if necessary;

4) check the impact of these modifications on blood glucose;

5) feel confident, safe and independent in managing his or her diabetes;

    and above all,

6) bring and keep blood glucose levels as close to normal as possible.

3. Why should the person with diabetes try to keep blood glucose levels as close to normal as possible?

A person with diabetes should try to keep blood glucose levels as close to normal as possible to prevent complications associated with diabetes.

Two major studies (one American study on type 1 diabetes and one British study on type 2 diabetes) have demonstrated that keeping blood glucose levels as close to normal as possible **significantly reduced the appearance and progression of complications due to diabetes:**

➤ **Retinopathy:**   21% to 76% decrease

➤ **Nephropathy:**   34% to 54% decrease

➤ **Neuropathy:**   40% to 60% decrease or improvement in existing neuropathy

4. How is blood glucose measured from the fingertip?

Blood glucose is measured from the fingertip with a glucose meter. The procedure involves two steps:

Preparing the materials and checking the reagent strips

1) **Wash your hands** with soapy water and dry them thoroughly. This reduces the risk of infection and makes it easier to take the blood sample. Alcohol

swabs are not recommended for home use because they can dry the skin, which may lead to cracked fingertips.

2) **Prepare the materials:** meter, test strip, lancing device, lancet, paper tissue.

3) **Insert the lancet into the lancing device** and set it. A lancet must never be used more than once. It should not be thrown directly into the trashcan; keep a rigid plastic container at hand for disposal. Never use a lancet or a lancing device that another person has already used.

4) Check the reagent strip container for the manufacturer's recommended expiration date.

5) If needed, write down on the container the date it was first opened in order to **keep track of the life expectancy of the strips.**

6) **Take out a test strip.** If the strip comes from a bottle, close it immediately.

Blood analysis and recording of data

1) Press the switch to start the device, if necessary.

2) Insert the test strip into the strip support on the device or automatically release a strip from the device.

3) Prick the **side of a finger tip** (use a different finger each time you take a blood sample).

4) Draw a **large drop of blood** by applying pressure on the finger while pointing it downwards. Do not "milk" the finger.

5) Place the **first drop of blood** on the reactive part of the strip or bring the reactive part of the strip into contact with the blood, depending on the device used.

6) Wait for the reading to be displayed.

7) **Write the result down** in the appropriate column of your glucose logbook.

5. Can other areas of the body be used to measure blood glucose?

Blood glucose can be measured with blood drawn from other areas of the body (**alternative sites**) such as the forearm, arm, palm of the hand, abdomen or thigh.

Currently, several glucose meters offer this option.

Results are generally comparable to glucose readings taken from the fingertip before a meal. However, there are restrictions on measuring blood glucose in this way. It is recommended that a blood glucose reading be taken from the fingertip in situations where blood glucose can fluctuate rapidly. This can occur:

1) during an episode of hypoglycemia;

2) during physical activity;

3) up to two hours after a meal;

4) very soon after an insulin injection;

5) during an illness.

6. Which glucose meters are currently available for purchase, and what are their features?

The chart on pages 50-51 contains a list of the latest glucose meters currently on the market, with some of their features (list revised as of July 1, 2004).

The cost of glucose meters can range anywhere from nothing to $300, depending on the model. Sales promotions or special offers are common, and certain devices are offered free with a trade-in.

Strips cost between $0.90 and $1.00 each. There are no special offers on strips.

7. What are the main causes of false glucose readings?

False readings occur when:

1) the glucose meter is dirty;

2) the glucose meter is calibrated incorrectly;

3) the user forgets to calibrate the meter, leaving out the calibration code for the current batch of reagent strips;

4) the strips have expired;

5) the strips have been exposed to humidity;

6) the strips have been exposed to extreme temperatures;

7) the drop of blood is too small;

8) the user's technique is faulty (e.g., withdrawing the finger from the meter before the "beep");

9) the glucose meter is inaccurate.

8. How can the accuracy of glucose meter results be verified?

The accuracy of results taken from a glucose meter should be verified annually. The **fasting blood glucose** level from a laboratory blood test should be compared with the level the patient obtains from the blood glucose meter. The blood glucose should be tested as usual, **within five minutes** of the blood sample.

The result of the **fasting blood glucose** reading taken from a blood glucose meter must **vary by less than 20%** from the blood glucose reading taken in the laboratory. For glucose readings less than or equal to 4.2 mmol/l, the difference should be smaller.

HOW CAN THE ACCURACY OF A GLUCOSE METER BE MEASURED?

Fasting

1) Have a nurse take a "fasting blood glucose" sample.
2) Take a glucose reading as usual, within five minutes of drawing the sample.
3) Write this down in the logbook and circle it.
4) Ask for the results of the analysis during the next visit to the doctor.
5) Calculate the accuracy of the meter (a difference of less than 20%).

	Example	Your results
Fasting blood glucose taken in the laboratory (from blood sample)	10 mmol/l	....
Blood glucose from meter (taken within 5 minutes)	9.2 mmol/l	....

Formula for calculating the accuracy of meter

$$\frac{\text{Glucose reading from meter} - \text{Fasting blood glucose}}{\text{Fasting blood glucose}} \times 100 = \text{Difference in \%}$$

$$(9.2 - 10.0) \div 10.0 \times 100 = 8.0\%$$

It is recommended that the result differ by less than 20%.

---

9. How often should blood glucose levels be measured?

Generally, a person with type 1 diabetes is advised to measure blood glucose at least three times a day at various intervals: **before each meal and before bedtime** (before a snack). Sometimes, the doctor responsible for treatment will advise the patient to measure blood glucose one or two hours after meals (generally timing the measurement from the first mouthful) and even during the night.

A person with non-insulin-dependent type 2 diabetes should measure blood glucose at least once a day, alternating between measurements before meals and before bedtime (before a snack). He or she may occasionally be directed to measure blood glucose one or two hours after meals (again generally timing the measurement from the first mouthful) and also during the night.

It is also recommended to measure blood glucose whenever unease or discomfort lead one to suspect hypoglycemia or hyperglycemia. In the case of illness, blood glucose should be measured more often.

Blood glucose levels should be tested more often whenever a lifestyle change occurs, whether in diet, medication or stress levels.

When engaging in physical activity, blood glucose should be measured before, during and after the activity.

10. What information should the person with diabetes record in the logbook to better self-monitor blood glucose?

To better self-monitor blood glucose, the diabetic person can write down the following information in the logbook:

1) the result and the date of the blood glucose reading (in the appropriate column relative to the meal; e.g., "Before lunch");

2) pertinent comments, such as the explanation for the **hypoglycemia** (a change in diet, physical activity, etc.);

3) the result of a **ketone bodies** reading from urine or blood, with the date and time (in the "Comments" column);

4) the name, dose and time of administration of **all prescribed antidiabetic medications**. Note every change and omission concerning medications (in the "Comments" column);

5) the quantity of carbohydrates ingested during meals and snacks;

6) the site of the **insulin** injection and, if applicable, the technique used, etc. (in the "Comments" column).

11. How should the person with diabetes record the information so that it is easy to analyze?

The information should be noted in the self-monitoring logbook. Each reading category should be written down in a clearly identified column:

1) in the first column, write down blood glucose readings taken **before the morning meal** in the course of a single week;

2) in the second column, write down blood glucose readings taken **after the morning meal** in the course of a single week;

3) in the appropriate columns that follow, write down **other blood glucose readings**, that is, those taken before and after the afternoon and evening meals, before bedtime (before a snack) and during the night;

4) **hypoglycemia** occurring outside the four usual periods of blood glucose readings should be written down at the next period (hypoglycemia occurring in the afternoon should be written down in the column preceding the evening meal);

5) unmeasured hypoglycemia should be given a reading of **2 mmol/l**;

6) the **weekly average** of glucose readings should be written down at the foot of each column (do not include the results of hypoglycemic correction when calculating the average). See the example indicated by two asterisks (**) in the table on the next page;

7) when calculating averages, do not include those readings associated with an exceptional, one-off, explainable situation; see the examples indicated by an asterisk (*) in the table on the next page;

8) pertinent comments should be written down in the appropriate columns.

Example of a self-monitoring logbook

Week beginning Sunday:					1 (day) 07 (month) 2004 (year)				
Day of the week	**Blood glucose measurements (mmol/l)**								**Comments**
	Breakfast		Lunch		Dinner		Bedtime		
	Before	After	Before	After	Before	After	Before snack		
Sunday	5.2		12.1						
Monday	7.1				8.1				
Tuesday	4.6						4.1		
Wednesday	9.3		10.4			12.3			
Thursday	5.5				7.2		6.7		
Friday	6.8				3.5*		16.6**		* Exercise ** Corrected hypoglycemia
Saturday	3.9		11.3		18.1*				* Stress
Average	6.1		11.3		7.7		5.4		

The average is calculated by adding up all the numbers in the same column and dividing the total by the number of measurements in that column.

Example: Average blood glucose before lunch:

$(12.1 + 10.4 + 11.3) \div 3 = 33.8 \div 3 = 11.3$

12. Besides blood glucose readings, will the doctor prescribe other tests to monitor blood glucose?

In addition to blood glucose readings, the doctor may prescribe blood tests to measure **glycosylated hemoglobin** or **fructosamine**. These two laboratory analyses show how well the diabetes has been managed:

➤ during the last two to three months, in the case of **glycosylated hemoglobin** (A1C);

➤ during the last two to three weeks, in the case of **fructosamine**.

LIST OF GLUCOSE METERS (REVISED AS OF JULY 1, 2004)

Name	Ascensia™ Elite™ XL	Ascensia™ Contour™	Ascensia™ Breeze™	BD Latitude™ and BD Logic™	OneTouch™ SureStep™	OneTouch™ Ultra™
Manufacturer	Bayer	Bayer	Bayer	BD	LifeScan	LifeScan
Measuring range (mmol/l)	1.1 to 33.3	0.6 to 33.3	0.6 to 33.3	1.1 to 33.3	0 to 27.8	1.1 to 33.3
Temperature range (°C)	10 to 40	10 to 40	10 to 40	15 to 39	10 to 35	6 to 44
Duration of analysis (sec)	30	15	30	5	30	5
Quantity of blood required (µL)	2	0.6	2.5 to 3.5	0.4	10	1.0
Possibility of adding a 2nd drop of blood	No	No	No	No	No	No
Cleaning required	No	No	No	No	Yes	No
Check strip	Yes	No	No	No	No	No
Calibration of test strips	Calibration strip in each box	Automatic	Automatic	Calibration code on each bottle	Calibration code on each bottle	Calibration code on each bottle
Life span of test strips	Date printed on packet	6 months (after opening)	Date printed on disk	3 months (after opening)	4 months (after opening)	3 months (after opening)
Test strips	Packaged individually	In a bottle (sensitive to humidity)	Disk of 10 strips	In a bottle (sensitive to humidity)	In a bottle (sensitive to humidity)	In a bottle (sensitive to humidity)
Lifespan of control solution, after opening	6 months	6 months	6 months	3 months	3 months	3 months
Memory (saved glucose tests)	120	240	100	250	150	150
Download to PC	Yes	Yes	Yes	Yes	Yes	Yes
Batteries and life expectancy	2 (lithium) 3 V no. CR2032 1,000 tests	2 (lithium) 3 V no. CR2032 1,000 tests	1 (lithium) 3 V no. CR2025 1,000 tests	1 (lithium) 3 V no. 2450 1,500 tests	2 (alkaline) AAA 1.5 V 1,000 tests	1 (lithium) 3 V no. CR2032 1,000 tests
Guarantee	5 years	5 years	5 years	3 years	6 years	6 years
Alternative sites	No	Yes	Yes	No	No	Yes
Lancing device	Microlet	Microlet	Microlet	BD Latitude	Penlet Plus	OneTouch UltraSoft
Lancets	Microlet 28 gauge	Microlet 28 gauge	Microlet 28 gauge	BD Latitude 33 gauge	UltraSoft 28 gauge	UltraSoft 28 gauge
Telephone support	1 800 268-7200	1 800 268-7200	1 800 268-7200	1 888 232-2737	1 800 663-5521	1 800 663-5521
Internet	www. ascensia.ca	www. ascensia.ca	www. ascensia.ca	www. bddiabetes.com	www. onetouch.ca	www. onetouch.ca

OneTouch™ UltraSmart™	InDuo™	Precision Xtra™ Glucose (G) and Ketone (K)	Precision Sof-Tact™	Accu-Chek™ Advantage™	Accu-Chek™ Compact™	FreeStyle™	FreeStyle™ Mini™
LifeScan	LifeScan/ Novo Nordisk	MediSense Abbott	MediSense Abbott	Roche Diagnostics	Roche Diagnostics	TheraSense Abbott	TheraSense Abbott
1.1 to 33.3	1.1 to 33.3	G: 1.1 to 27.8 K: 0 to 6.0	1.7 to 25	0.6 to 33.3	0.6 to 33.3	1.1 to 27.8	1.1 to 27.8
6 to 44	6 to 44	15 to 40	18 to 30	14 to 40	10 to 40	5 to 40	5 to 40
5	5	G: 10 K: 30	20	26	8	15	7
1.0	1.0	G: 1.5 K: 5.0	2.5	4	1.5	0.3	0.3
No	No	Yes (within next 30 sec.)	No	Yes (within next 15 sec.)	Yes (within next 25 sec.)	Yes (within next 60 sec.)	Yes (within next 60 sec.)
No	No	No	Yes	No	Yes	No	No
No	No	Yes (available from the manufacturer)	Yes (available from the manufacturer)	No	No	No	No
Calibration code on each bottle	Calibration code on each bottle	Calibration strip in each box	Calibration strip in each box	Calibration chip in each box	Automatic	Calibration code on each bottle	Calibration code on each bottle
3 months (after opening)	3 months (after opening)	Date printed on packet	Date printed on packet	Date printed on bottle	3 months (after use of cartridge)	Date printed on bottle	Date printed on bottle
In a bottle (sensitive to humidity)	In a bottle (sensitive to humidity)	Packaged individually	Packaged individually	In a bottle	Cartridge of 17 strips	In a bottle	In a bottle
3 months	3 months	3 months	3 months	3 months	3 months	3 months	3 months
3,000	150	450	450	480	100	250	250
Yes	Yes	Yes	Yes	Yes	Yes	Yes	Yes
2 (alkaline) AAA 1.5 V 540 tests	1 (lithium) 3 V no. CR2032 1,000 tests	2 (alkaline) AAA, 1.5 V 1,000 tests	1 (alkaline) 9 V 365 tests	1 (lithium) 3 V no. CR2032 1,000 tests	2 (alkaline) AAA 1.5 V 500 tests	2 (alkaline) AAA 1.5 V 1,000 tests	2 (lithium) 3 V no. CR2032 500 tests
3 years	3 years	4 years	4 years	5 years	5 years	5 years	5 years
Yes	Yes	No	Yes	No	Yes	Yes	Yes
OneTouch UltraSoft	OneTouch UltraSoft	MediSense	Integrated	SoftClix	SoftClix	FreeStyle	FreeStyle
UltraSoft 28 gauge	UltraSoft 28 gauge	Precision 28 gauge	Ultra TLC 28 gauge	SoftClix Select 28 gauge	SoftClix Select 28 gauge	FreeStyle 25 gauge	FreeStyle 25 gauge
1 800 663-5521	1 800 663-5521	1 800 461-8481	1 800 461-8481	1 800 363-7949	1 800 363-7949	1 888 519-6890	1 888 519-6890
www. onetouch.ca	www. induo.com	www.medisense. com	www.medisense. com	www. accu-chek.com	www. accu-chek.com	www. therasense.com	www. therasense.com

CHAPTER 5

Measuring Ketone Bodies

1. What are ketone bodies?

Ketone bodies are the **by-products of the breakdown of body fat**.

2. What does an increase of ketone bodies in the blood mean?

An increase of ketone bodies in the blood indicates that the person with diabetes is using **fat** reserves stored in the body instead of glucose. This is due to a **lack of insulin**.

Without insulin, the cells of the body cannot use glucose in the blood. When this happens, the body will use energy stored in the form of fat. The breakdown of fat produces **ketone bodies**. These ketone bodies are acids which may lead to **diabetic ketoacidosis**.

Excess ketone bodies in the blood are eliminated into the urine. It is therefore possible to measure excess ketone bodies in either blood or urine.

3.   Why must a person with diabetes check for excess ketone bodies in the blood or urine?

A person with diabetes—especially type 1—must check for excess ketone bodies in the blood or urine **because an excess indicates that the diabetes is poorly managed** and that there is a risk of diabetic ketoacidosis. Ketoacidosis can lead to coma. In some cases, a doctor may recommend this monitoring procedure to people with type 2 diabetes.

4.   When do people with diabetes have to check for excess ketone bodies in their blood or urine?

People with diabetes must check for the presence of ketone bodies in their blood or urine **when their blood glucose is higher than 14 mmol/l or when a doctor recommends it.**

They must continue performing this test—in addition to measuring blood glucose four times a day or more often if necessary—until there are no excess **ketone bodies** in the blood or urine and **blood glucose** is back to **normal.**

They must also perform this test when experiencing the following symptoms:

1)   intense or excessive thirst;

2)   abdominal pain;

3)   excessive tiredness or drowsiness;

4)   nausea and vomiting.

5.   What must a person with diabetes do when there are excess ketone bodies in the blood or urine?

A person with diabetes who finds excess ketone bodies in the blood or urine must:

1) **drink 250 ml** of water hourly to help eliminate the ketone bodies through the urine;

2) **take supplemental doses of Humalog®, NovoRapid®, Humulin® or Novolin® ge Toronto insulin,** following the recommendations of the doctor responsible for treatment (see chapter 21 on hyperglycemic emergencies);

3) call a doctor or go to the emergency department immediately if an excess of ketone bodies in the blood or urine persists despite treatment, and if the following symptoms appear:

   ➤ abdominal pain;

   ➤ excessive tiredness or drowsiness;

   ➤ nausea and vomiting.

6. How is the presence of ketone bodies measured in urine?

Ketone bodies in urine are measured with a reagent strip.

Preparing the materials

1) Gather the materials: **Ketostix®** reagent strips, a dry and clean container and a chronometer.

2) Check the manufacturer's expiry date on the reagent strip container. Mark the container with the date it was first opened. It must be discarded **six months** after being opened.

   ➤ Ketostix® reagent strips must be stored at room temperature (between 18ºC and 25ºC).

3) Collect a **fresh** urine sample for analysis:

   ➤ first, empty the bladder completely and discard the urine;

   ➤ drink one or two glasses of water;

   ➤ next, urinate into a dry, clean container.

4)   Take a reagent strip from the container and close it **immediately**.

➤   Compare the colour of the reagent strip to the colour chart on the container to ensure that the strip has not changed colour, which could provide a false result.

Testing the urine sample with the reagent strip

1)   Dip the reactive part of the strip into the fresh urine sample and remove it right away.

2)   Use the edge of the container to help the remaining fluid drain off the strip and start the timer.

Reading the results and writing them down

1)   After **exactly 15 seconds**, place the reagent strip next to the colour chart on the strip container and compare the result under a bright light.

2)   Write down the result in your glucose self-monitoring logbook.

Negative	Trace	Small	Moderate	Large
0	0.5 mmol/l	1.5 mmol/l	4 mmol/l	8 mmol/l to 16 mmol/l

Reagent strips that simultaneously measure glucose and ketone bodies in the urine (e.g., Keto-Diastix®, Chemstrip® u G/K) are also available.

7.   How is the level of ketone bodies measured from a fingertip blood sample?

Ketone bodies in the blood are measured with a ketone meter.

Preparing the materials

1) Gather the materials: **Precision Xtra®** meter, test strips for measuring ketosis (ketone bodies), lancing device, lancet.

2) Check the expiry date on the reagent strip envelope.

3) Insert the ketone calibrator into the Precision Xtra® meter. The code on the screen must match the code on the strip.

4) Insert the ketone strip into the Precision Xtra® meter.

Applying the blood sample to the reagent strip

1) Prick the fingertip using the lancing device (holder).

2) Apply a drop of blood to the target area of the strip.

Reading the result and writing it down

1) Wait 30 seconds for the result to appear on the screen.

2) Write down the result in the self-monitoring logbook.

Negative	Trace	Small	Moderate	Large
0	Less than 0.6 mmol/l	0.6 mmol/l to 1.5 mmol/l	1.5 mmol/l to 3 mmol/l	More than 3 mmol/l

CHAPTER 6

Eating Well

1. Why is it important for a diabetic person to eat well?

Eating well, along with regular exercise and abstention from smoking, is part of a wholesome routine that promotes good health and controls the disease more effectively.

There are no "forbidden foods" and there is no "diabetic diet". Rather, the focus is on choosing foods wisely and managing portion sizes. The diet of a diabetic person should be satisfying, varied and balanced rather than restrictive or punitive.

A treatment regimen may consist solely of a dietary plan or it may include oral antidiabetic medications and insulin. Either way, healthy eating is essential.

2. Why is eating well important for a diabetic person?

Eating well offers a number of advantages for a person with diabetes. A healthy diet:

1) promotes better control of:

- blood glucose;
- weight;
- blood pressure;
- fat levels in blood;

2)   satisfies the body's energy, vitamin and mineral requirements;

3)   promotes well-being.

3.   What does it mean to eat well?

Eating well means choosing **quality foods,** such as:

1)   dark green or orange vegetables and orange fruits as often as possible;

2)   whole grain or enriched cereal products, low-fat milk products, lean meat and poultry, fish and legumes;

3)   a wide variety of foods each day.

Eating well also means choosing the **right quantity or servings** for your energy needs. A person's dietary requirements are a function of age, body build, gender and activity level.

Finally, eating well means:

1)   taking the time to eat, in other words, setting aside a period reserved just for eating;

2)   eating slowly, in other words, taking 15 to 20 minutes or more for a meal from beginning to end;

3)   paying attention to the body's signals of hunger and satiety, that is, recognizing when you have eaten enough.

4.   How can eating well help in managing blood glucose?

Of all the food groups, carbohydrates have the greatest influence on blood glucose levels. A diabetic person will maintain better control of blood glucose if:

1) meals are taken at regular hours, that is, at the same time from day to day;

2) nutrition is evenly spread over at least three meals, spaced about four to six hours apart;

3) carbohydrates are evenly spread over three meals rather than consumed once a day (such as during the evening meal);

4) no meal is skipped;

5) the carbohydrate content of each meal is consistent from one day to the next;

6) the carbohydrate content consumed during and, if necessary, between meals corresponds to one's energy needs. Eating too many carbohydrates can be detrimental to the effective control of blood glucose.

5. How can eating well help with weight control?

Eating well can help some people lose weight when they choose **foods containing fewer calories.**

For overweight people, losing between 5% and 10% of excess weight may be enough to improve control of blood glucose levels, blood pressure and fat levels in blood.

6. How can eating well help control fat levels in blood?

Choosing **leaner foods** containing higher quality fats can help control fat levels in blood. Higher fat levels in blood increase the risk of cardiovascular diseases.

7.   How can eating well help manage blood pressure?

Eating **fresh foods** as often as possible can help lower blood pressure, since they are not processed and therefore generally contain less salt than canned or delicatessen foods. Furthermore, fresh fruit and vegetables are rich in potassium, which helps lower blood pressure. Moderate alcohol consumption (two drinks a day or fewer) is also recommended.

8.   How can eating well be pleasurable?

Eating well should be one of life's pleasures. The need for a meal plan does not mean one must avoid foods that delight the senses of sight, smell and taste. But above all, eating well can produce a **feeling of well-being.** Some people discover that feeling better becomes their primary motivation to develop better habits and maintain a healthy lifestyle.

9.   Does eating well mean avoiding cold cuts, French fries, chips and pastries?

These foods are acceptable and can be part of a healthy diet. While it is true that they are often high in fat, sugar, and calories, including them on occasion in a meal plan is a matter of personal choice. Excluding them is also an option, especially if weight loss is the goal. However, this could also be a mistake, since it may have a boomerang effect, creating an obsession for these types of food and thus leading to overindulgence.

10. How can we develop better nutritional habits when a change in diet is necessary?

Here are several suggestions for improving eating habits:

1)   Set clear, measurable and realistic goals.

2) Go about it gradually, one modification at a time. Small changes can make a big difference.

3) Create a meal plan with the help of a dietician.

4) Choose satisfying foods. This will help you prevent slips and maintain control over diabetes.

5) Replace food rewards with other treats. For example, buy a book or CD, or take a relaxing bath to pamper yourself.

11. What is a meal plan?

A meal plan is a personalized guide for a diabetic person who wants to eat well. It promotes a diet rich in a wide variety of foods from the different food groups. It also helps determine the quantity and quality of foods consumed, according to a personalized timetable. The meal plan follows to dietary recommendations, helping you stay healthy, and is a complement to medications for the treatment of diabetes and other ailments associated with it.

It puts the accent on **quality foods** and healthy choices. It is built on the six food groups:

➤ starches;

➤ fruits;

➤ vegetables;

➤ milk;

➤ meat and alternatives;

➤ fats.

It outlines **quantities or servings appropriate** to the individual's energy needs. It specifies the recommended carbohydrate content for each meal and snack, as well as the number of servings of meat or meat substitutes and fats.

The plan can serve as the model for your daily meals. It helps standardize the quantities and servings of food consumed from one day to the next, promoting better control of blood glucose levels while acknowledging the importance of a varied diet.

People with diabetes are strongly advised to eat at regular hours and to keep these consistent from day to day. This is particularly important for a person with diabetes taking oral antidiabetic insulin stimulants (e.g., Diabeta®) or insulin because it can help reduce major fluctuations in blood glucose levels, such as hyperglycemia or hypoglycemia.

12. Are snacks necessary?

Snacking, in general, is not necessary, but including snacks in your meal plan can help you spread out your carbohydrates intake evenly over the course of a day.

Insulin users are sometimes advised to have a snack containing carbohydrates at night, as late as possible.

CHAPTER 7

Carbohydrates: Knowing How to Recognize Them

1. Should carbohydrates be eaten even though they raise blood glucose levels?

Carbohydrates are an essential energy source for the body. It is therefore appropriate and necessary to consume foods containing carbohydrates at every meal, even though they may raise blood glucose. Carbohydrates should provide half of a person's energy requirements. For example, if a person needs to consume 1,800 calories per day, half of them (900 calories) should come from carbohydrates.

2. What are dietary carbohydrates?

Dietary carbohydrates are often refered to as "sugars" in everyday speech. However, in this book, "sugar" refers exclusively to white sugar, saccharose or sucrose.

There are several types of dietary carbohydrates:

1) glucose;

2) fructose;

3) saccharose (sucrose);

4) lactose;

5) polyols such as sorbitol, mannitol, xylitol, lactitol, isomalt, etc.;

6) starches;

7) dietary fibre.

3. What information do food product labels provide on carbohydrate content?

The carbohydrate content listed on food product labels includes sugars, starches and dietary fibre. In this context, the term "sugars" refers to glucose, fructose, saccharose (sucrose) and lactose, among others. These sugars occur naturally in some foods; they can also be added to specific products. "Sugar alcohols" are sometimes listed as well; this term refers to polyols such as sorbitol, mannitol, xylitol, isomalt, maltitol and lactitol.

4. Which foods contain carbohydrates?

Of the six food groups, only two — meat and its substitutes and fats — contain little or no carbohydrates.

Four of the food groups contain carbohydrates. They are starches, fruits, vegetables and milk.

➤ **Starches, fruits and milk:**

Servings from these three groups provide an average of 15 g of carbohydrates or the equivalent of 3 tsp. of sugar. For example:

Foods	One serving
Starches	
Bread	1 slice weighing 30 g
Cooked spaghetti	125 ml ($^1/2$ cup)
Rusks	2
Fruits	
Banana	$^1/2$ (small)
Grapes	15
Orange juice	125 ml ($^1/2$ cup)
Milk	
Milk	250 ml (1 cup)
Plain yogourt	175 ml ($^3/4$ cup)

➤ **Vegetables:**

Most raw and cooked vegetables contain little in the way of carbohydrates: one serving of vegetables contains an average of 5 g of carbohydrates, or the equivalent of 1 tsp. of sugar. Therefore, these foods will have little effect on blood glucose, unless they are consumed in large quantities in one sitting (three servings providing 15 g of carbohydrates).

5. How can carbohydrate content be determined?

There are different methods of measuring the carbohydrate content of foods. The most common are:

1) Carbohydrate equivalents or food group exchange system:

The system of equivalents or food group exchange is mainly used by people with diabetes who are following a dietary regimen, or by those taking oral antidiabetic medications or insulin combined with fixed amounts of carbohydrates. It allows the carbohydrate content of meals to be assessed in terms of equivalent 15 g servings of carbohydrates.

This method is used by Diabetes Québec and the American Diabetes Association (ADA). The Canadian Diabetes Association (CDA) uses a system with different food groupings and serving sizes. The chart below presents the main differences between the systems. The CDA system is presently under revision and will soon more closely resemble the one used by Diabetes Québec and the ADA.

CARBOHYDRATE CONTENT FOR ONE SERVING		
Food groups containing carbohydrates	**Methods recommended by**	
	ADA and Diabetes Québec	*ACD*
Milk	12 g to 15 g (250 ml)	6 g (125 ml)
Vegetables	0 g to 5 g	—
Fruits	15 g	—
Vegetables and fruits	—	10 g
Starches	15 g	15 g
Other carbohydrates	Read label	10 g

Example: one apple serving

	Methods recommended by	
	ADA and Diabetes Québec	*ACD*
One apple serving is equivalent to:	1 small weighing 100 g	1/2 medium weighing 75 g
Carbohydrate content in a serving of fruit:	15 g	10 g

To simplify the explanation given here of these systems, all foods containing carbohydrates (excluding vegetables) are grouped in such a way that any given serving provides approximately 15 g of carbohydrates (also equivalent to 15 ml or 3 tsp. of sugar). Therefore, the basic unit is 15 g of carbohydrates.

2) Carbohydrate counting:

People with diabetes who inject short-acting insulin according to a varied carbohydrate intake should learn to count the total carbohydrate content of their meals as precisely as possible in order to optimize their treatment.

A sugar cube (or a teaspoon or packet of sugar) is often used as a basic unit to help people visualize the carbohydrate content of foods. Using this model, 5 g of carbohydrates are equivalent to 1 cube (or 1 tsp. or 1 packet) of sugar.

6. Can meals include foods that are not part of the six food groups (for example, pastries, jams, or soft drinks)?

Foods containing fewer than 3 g of carbohydrates per serving need not be included in the meal's carbohydrate total, provided that they are eaten one serving at a time and that the servings are adequately spaced throughout the day.

For example:

The 2.5 g carbohydrate content of 10 ml or 2 tsp. of light fruit jam is not usually added to the carbohydrate tally for breakfast.

Other foods containing 3 g of carbohydrates or more per serving may be eaten on an occasional basis, as long as one keeps track of their carbohydrate content, which must be counted in order to avoid exceeding the amount required per meal.

Pastries, pies, cookies, ice cream, chocolate, chips, crackers, etc., contain fats as well as carbohydrates. Therefore, their caloric content is quite high. Those who are weight-conscious should be aware that these foods can contribute to weight gain.

7. How can we find out about the carbohydrate content of foods?

There are several ways to find out about the carbohydrate content of the foods we consume.

1) Product labels:

The main way to find out about the carbohydrate content of foods is to read the list of nutritional values on the product label.

2) Food composition tables:

Health Canada publishes a useful table called "Nutrient Value of Some Common Foods" (2003). It is available in bookstores or on the Health Canada web site.

3) Fast-food restaurants:

Some restaurants provide nutritional information about the foods they serve. Be sure to ask.

4) Recipe books:

Many recipe books list the nutritional value of their recipes.

5) The list of food exchanges:

Provided by your dietician, this list is an excellent resource for nutritional information. In addition, the list published by the ministère de la Santé et des Services sociaux du Québec (Quebec's Minister of Health) in conjunction with Diabetes Québec (*Meal Planning for People with Diabetes*) is also highly recommended.

8. What amount of carbohydrates can you eat per day?

Total daily carbohydrate intake is determined by energy (or caloric) needs, which are evaluated according to a person's size, weight, gender, age and physical activity.

On average, carbohydrates should meet half of a person's caloric needs. The rest should be provided by proteins, fats and alcohol.

To maintain optimal body function, a person should consume more than 100 g of carbohydrates a day. Generally, the amount should fall between 200 g and 300 g per day.

9. Should the same quantity of carbohydrates be eaten every day?

It depends on the individual's treatment regimen.

1) **People with diabetes whose treatment consists solely of a dietary regimen or a diet combined with a fixed medical treatment** (either oral antidiabetic medications or insulin) should eat the same quantity of carbohydrates at every meal and schedule meals at regular hours.

   The total carbohydrate intake should be spread out over the course of the day. This will help:

   ➤ people whose treatment consists solely of a dietary regimen or a diet combined with oral antidiabetic medication to avoid a blood glucose spike after meals;

   ➤ people who use insulin to ensure that carbohydrate consumption coincides with insulin action.

2) **People who count carbohydrates and inject insulin according to the amount of carbohydrates ingested** may vary their carbohydrate consumption from day to day. Having a balanced meal should remain a priority because it is vital to good health and because overeating brings with it the risk of weight gain.

10. Why is it beneficial to incorporate fibre-rich foods in the diet?

Fibre-rich foods are forms of carbohydrates. They are not digested in the small intestine and arrive intact in the large intestine. This explains why fibre does not raise blood glucose levels.

Some sources of fibre
Oatmeal and wheat flour
Fruits
Whole grains
Vegetables
Legumes
Nuts
Oat and wheat bran

Eating a wide variety of fibre rich foods in fibre is recommended since they are also a good source of vitamins and minerals. Moreover, fibre helps:

1) **control blood glucose:** large amounts of fibre help some people with diabetes control blood glucose;

2) **control constipation:** fibre increases stool volume and promotes a healthy colon (large intestine);

3) **control blood cholesterol:** large amounts of fibre help some people with diabetes lower blood cholesterol;

4) **control weight:** foods rich in fibre have minimal energy value but still leave you feeling full.

CHAPTER 8

Fats: Making Good Choices

1. Why should we eat less fat?

Eating less fat helps us to control fat levels in our blood. These are the different existing fats:

➡ triglycerides;

➡ total cholesterol;

➡ HDL-cholesterol (good cholesterol);

➡ LDL-cholesterol (bad cholesterol).

People with diabetes are at significant risk of developing cardiovascular diseases. If a person with diabetes has high amounts of triglycerides and bad cholesterol in his or her blood, this risk is even higher.

Limiting fat consumption also helps control weight.

2. How can fat consumption lead to weight gain?

If a gram of carbohydrate or protein contains four calories, a gram of fat contains nine calories (that is, more than the double of the first number).

➤ 5 ml or 1 tsp. of sugar (5 g of carbohydrates) contains 20 calories, while

➤ 5 ml or 1 tsp. of oil (5 g of fat) contains about 45 calories.

3. What is the recommended daily fat consumption for a healthy diet?

The allowance of calories we consume in one day should be spread out as follows:

➤ 30% to 35% should come from fats ($\leq$ 10% from trans or saturated fats and between 0.6% and 1.2% from alpha-linolenic acid);

➤ 50% to 55% from carbohydrates (from a variety of sources);

➤ 15% from proteins (from a variety of sources).

4. Should a person with diabetes count fats the way he or she counts carbohydrates?

Not necessarily. In general, making healthier choices such as eating smaller portions of meat or choosing leaner cheese will be enough to reduce the amount of fat that a person consumes. We eat too much fat and we often eat it on impulse, because fatty foods taste so irresistibly delicious. Fat content gives flavour to food, making dishes containing it more attractive than others foods.

5. Which foods contain fats?

The following foods contain either visible or hidden fats:

Visible fats	Hidden fats
Oils	Meats and deli meats
Butter	Higher-fat fish (mackerel and sardines, among others)
Margarine	Mayonnaise
Lard	Sauces (including gravies and cream or cheese based sauces)
Vegetable fats	
Meats	Certain prepared dishes
	Nuts and grains
	Baked goods, pastries, and sweets

6. Which fats occur naturally in foods?

There are three:

1) saturated fats, which are usually of animal origin;

2) cholesterol, which is always of animal origin;

3) unsaturated fats, which are mainly of vegetable origin; these may be monounsaturated or polyunsaturated.

No food consists solely of one type of fat. Fats are classified according to the predominant type of fat present.

For example:

Sunflower oil, which is very high in polyunsaturated fats, also contains small quantities of saturated and monounsaturated fats. Therefore, it is classified as a source of polyunsaturated fats.

7. What are trans or hydrogenated fats, such as those found in certain margarines and vegetable shortenings?

These are fats produced by the food industry, that are not found in natural or unprocessed foods. Trans and hydrogenated fats are made from unsaturated fats, especially oils, which have been processed. This process converts oils from a liquid to a solid state. Regular consumption of these fats increases the risk of cardiovascular diseases.

Partially hydrogenated margarine and vegetable shortening are examples of this.

8. Why should we choose fats wisely?

People who have abnormal levels of fat in their blood or who have a history of high cholesterol should be aware of the different types of fats in foods. While some fats can be detrimental to our health, others can have positive, healthful effects when consumed in moderation.

Negative effects:

	Triglycerides	Total cholesterol	HDL-cholesterol	LDL-cholesterol
Cholesterol		↑		↑
Saturated fats		↑	↓	↑
Trans fatty acids or hydrogenated fats		↑	↓	↑

↑ increase ↓ decrease

Positive effects:

	Triglycerides	Total cholesterol	HDL-cholesterol	LDL-cholesterol
Monounsaturated fats	=	↓	↑ or =	↓
Polyunsaturated omega-3 fats	↓ or =	=	↑ or =	↑ or =

↑ increase   ↓ decrease   = no change

As we can see, some types of fats are better for our heart and blood vessels than others. Foods containing **monounsaturated and polyunsaturated** fats should be chosen over those containing saturated fats, trans or hydrogenated fats and cholesterol.

9. Why is it necessary to eat fats if they may have negative effects?

Fats are part of a balanced diet, just like carbohydrates and proteins. They contain essential fatty acids. These fatty acids carry fat-soluble vitamins and hormones, and are vital to various body processes.

10. What kinds of fats do we eat and in which foods are they found?

SATURATED FATS	
Animal origin[*]	**Vegetable origin**
Butter	Coconut or copra oil
Cream, ice cream	Palm oil
Cheese	Palm kernel oil
Whole milk (3.25% m.f.)	Coconut
Lard	
Eggs	
Suet	
Meats	
Poultry and poultry skin	

[*] These foods also contain cholesterol.

UNSATURATED FATS	
Monounsaturated	**Polyunsaturated**
Almonds	Pumpkin seeds
Peanuts	Linseed
Avocados	Sunflower seeds
Sesame seeds	Borage oil
Peanut oil	Safflower oil
Canola oil	Pumpkin oil
Olive oil	Linseed oil
Hazelnut oil	Corn oil
Sesame oil	Walnut oil
Hazelnuts	Grapeseed oil
Cashew nuts	Soya oil
Brazil nuts	Sunflower oil
Olives	Evening primrose oil
Pecans	Walnuts
Pistachios	Pine nuts
	Higher-fat fish (salmon, mackerel, etc.)

SATURATED FATS
Monounsaturated and polyunsaturated
Soft non-hydrogenated margarine (e.g. Becel®, Crystal®, Lactantia®, Nuvel®, Olivina®, etc.)

TRANS OR HYDROGENATED FATS OF VEGETABLE ORIGIN	
Hydrogenated vegetable oil	Soft margarine
Hard margarine	Vegetable oil shortening

11. How can we eat less fat and lower our consumption of trans or hydrogenated fats?

It is important to control our intake of fat.

To help us eat less fat, it is useful to know that:

1) all fats have comparable energy values: 5 ml (or 1 tsp.) of oil, butter or margarine contain 40 to 45 calories;

2) no oil is low-fat, even if it is " light."

To eat less fat, we can:

1) develop the habit of measuring oils, butter, and margarine with a teaspoon or a tablespoon;

2) choose leaner meat and poultry, and trim visible fat before cooking;

3) eat reasonably sized portions of meat;

4) include more fish in our diet – eat fish at least two or three times a week;

5) eat less cheese or choose fresh and leaner cheeses (e.g., cottage cheese). Cheese with over 20% fat contains two to three times more fat than an equivalent portion of meat;

6)   choose partially skimmed or skimmed milk (1% m.f. or 2% m.f.) instead of whole milk (3.25% m.f.);

7)   reduce our daily consumption of fatty foods such as butter and cream sauces, pastries, pre-packaged baked goods, sweets, croissants, etc.

12.   Which cooking methods can lower fat content?

When cooking, use methods that require the least fat possible.

Cooking method	Foods
Boiling	Boiled beef, boiled chicken
Steaming	Vegetables, fish, pressure-cooked rice
Roasting, baking or microwaving	Poultry, roasts (beef, pork, chicken, lamb, veal), fish, fruit, casseroles
Double-boiler cooking	Scrambled eggs
Stewing/Slow cooking	Mixed plate cooked in clay, casserole or pressure cooker
Grilling	Poultry, vegetables, higher-fat fish such as salmon, grilled in cast-iron cookware, in the oven or on the barbecue
Frying	Non-stick frying pan for eggs, omelettes and sliced meat
En papillote[1]	Fish, lean meat, vegetables, fruit
Simmering or braising	Meat
Using coarse salt (*au gros sel*)[2]	Fish, chicken

---

[1] A healthful and delicious French cooking method in which certain foods are wrapped in parchment paper or tinfoil and baked briefly.

[2] Heat the coarse salt (*gros sel*) in the oven between two aluminum cooking sheets for 30 minutes at 500 °F (260 °C). Remove the salt from the oven and put in the chicken or fish. Allow to cook 30 minutes at 350 °F (175 °C).

13. Are there foods that can help lower fat levels in blood?

Yes, certain food components can lower fat levels in blood, namely vegetable phytosterols, omega-3 fatty acids and soluble fibre.

1) **Vegetable phytosterols** (or sterols/stanols) have a beneficial effect on fat levels in blood. They are believed to prevent the absorption of cholesterol in the intestine. As a result, they reduce the amount of bad cholesterol in the blood. To obtain this result, the recommended daily consumption is 2 to 3 g of vegetable sterols, which are found mainly in vegetable oils, nuts and seeds, as well as in whole grains.

2) **Omega-3 fatty acids** help promote a healthy cardiovascular system. These heart-friendly nutrients are found in foods of both vegetable and animal origin. Their recommended daily intake is 1.1 g for women and 1.6 g for men. The following chart offers several examples of dietary, sources of omega-3 fatty acids, as well as their total fatty acid content per serving.

SOURCES OF OMEGA-3 FATTY ACIDS	
Foods	**Total quantities (g)**
Omega-3 milk (250 ml or 1 cup)	0.3
Omega-3 eggs* (100 g or 2 eggs)	0.8
Canned tuna (100 g or 3 oz.)	0.94
Soya oil (15 ml or 3 tsp.)	0.94
Walnuts (30 ml or 6 tsp.)	1.15
Canola oil (15 ml or 3 tsp.)	1.29
Mackerel (100 g or 3 oz.)	1.43
Ground linseed (10 ml or 2 tsp.)	1.45
Herring (100 g or 3 oz.)	2.22
Linseed oil (15 ml or 3 tsp.)	7.36

* Eggs from hens raised on linseed feed

Because omega-3 fatty acids found in fish are better for us than those found in foods of vegetable origin, two to three servings of fish per week are recommended.

3) Soluble fibre also has a beneficial effect on bad cholesterol. The recommended daily intake is from 10 and 25 g. The following foods provide a minimum of 3 g of soluble fibre per serving:

Fibre source	Quantity
All Bran® bran buds	75 ml (^{1}/3 cup)
Psyllium husks or powder	5 ml (1 tsp)
Metamucil®	15 ml (1 tbsp)
Cooked oat bran or porridge	250 ml (1 cup)
Red kidney beans	125 ml (^{1}/2 cup)
Ground linseed	75 ml (^{1}/3 cup)
Roasted soy seeds	75 ml (^{1}/3 cup)
Canned artichoke hearts	2

14. Are there other strategies to lower the fat levels in our blood?

The following factors may help to control and maintain healthy levels of fat in the blood:

	Triglycerides	Total cholesterol	HDL-cholesterol	LDL-cholesterol
Increasing physical activity	↓	↓	↑ or =	↓
Losing weight	↓			
Quitting smoking[3]	↓	↓	↑	↓

↑ increase   ↓ decrease   = no change

[3] The effect of smoking observed on fat levels in the blood may be linked to other factors associated with quitting smoking.

CHAPTER 9

Knowing How to Read Food Labels

1. What information is found on prepackaged food labels?

The following nutritional information is found on prepackaged food labels:

1) the nutrition information chart;

2) the list of ingredients;

3) the nutritional claims for the product.

2. What information does the nutrition information chart provide?

The nutrition information chart on a prepackaged food label provides information for a specified quantity of food:

1) the caloric value of the food in the given serving;

2) the content of 13 specific nutrients in the given serving;

3) the percentage of recommended daily intake (RDI).

Nutrition information per 125 ml (87 g)			
Content			% daily value
Calories	80		
Fat	0,5 g		1%
Saturated 0 g			
+ Trans	**0%**		
Cholesterol	0 mg		0%
Sodium	0 mg		0%
Carbohydrate	18 g		6%
Dietary fibres 2 g			8%
Sugars 2 g			
Protein 3 g			
Vitamin A	2%	Vitamin C	10%
Calcium	0%	Iron	2%

3.   What information is provided by the list of ingredients?

This list includes all the ingredients used in a specific food. They are sorted in descending order of weight, with those used in the largest quantities (the heaviest ingredients) listed first.

4.   What kinds of nutritional claims can manufacturers make?

A manufacturer can make two sorts of nutritional claims:

1) **claims regarding nutrient content:** these are related to the amount of nutrients present in the food;

2) **claims regarding health:** these must be authorized, and bring out the relationship between the food and a specific disease, ailment or health condition (cholesterol, cavities, osteoporosis, hypertension, cardiovascular diseases).

5. **Which nutritional claims regarding nutrient content can be found on a label?**

The following chart shows several examples of claims concerning nutritional information that can be found on food product labels, as well as the conditions under which these claims can be made.

Claims	Conditions – amount to be specified in conjunction with the food and serving size indicated on label
Energy	
"Calorie-reduced"	At least 25% calorie-reduced
"Low in calories"	No more than 40 calories
"Calorie-free"	Less than 5 calories
Fats	
"Fat-free"	Less than 0.5 g of fat
"Low-fat"	No more than 3 g of fat
"Low in saturated fats"	No more than 2 g of saturated fat and trans fat and no more than 15% of total calories derived from saturated fat and trans fat
"No trans fatty acids"	Less than 0.2 g of trans fatty acids and "low in saturated fats"
Cholesterol	
"No cholesterol"	Less than 2 mg of cholesterol

When the term "light" is used on a product, the manufacturer's label must indicate what makes the food "light". If the term "light" refers to the nutritional value of the food, it is to be used only for food products with a reduced amount of calories or lipids (fats).

6.   Which health claims are permitted on food labels?

Only scientifically proven health claims are authorized to appear on food labels. Here is the list:

> ➤ decreased sodium content and increased potassium content of a food can help lower arterial hypertension (blood pressure);

> ➤ increased calcium and vitamin D content of a food can help prevent osteoporosis;

> ➤ decreased saturated fat and trans or hydrogenated fat content of a food can help prevent cardiovascular diseases;

> ➤ increased consumption of fruit and vegetables can help prevent certain types of cancer;

> ➤ decreased carbohydrate content in candies, gum or breath fresheners can help to prevent cavities.

7.   What are sugar substitutes?

Sugar substitutes are substances that replace table sugar (saccharose or sucrose) and that are used to sweeten foods. Some of these substitutes add calories or carbohydrates while others do not. For that reason, sugar substitutes are described as **nutritive** or **non-nutritive**. The calories or carbohydrates added by nutritive sweeteners must be included in the meal plan and may affect blood glucose levels to different degrees. Non-nutritive sweeteners that provide no energy have little effect on blood glucose.

8.   Which nutritive sugar substitutes are found in foods?

The following chart lists the various nutritive sugar substitutes and their properties.

Nutritive substitutes	Energy (calories/g)	Sweetening power (%)*	Comments
Fructose	4	120-170	May increase triglycerides and cholesterol. Lower blood glucose reaction than sugar. Daily consumption of 60 g not recommended for people with diabetes.
Sorbitol	2.6	50-70	Does not cause cavities. Daily dose of 10 g may cause gastrointestinal discomfort. Lower blood glucose reaction than sugar.
Mannitol	1.6	50-70	Does not cause cavities. Daily dose of 10 g may cause gastrointestinal discomfort. Lower blood glucose reaction than sugar.
Xylitol	2.4	100	Does not cause cavities. Lower blood glucose reaction than sugar.
Lactilol	2	30-40	Does not cause cavities. Lower blood glucose reaction than sugar.
Isomalt	2	45-65	Does not cause cavities. Lower blood glucose reaction than sugar.
Maltitol	3	90	Does not cause cavities. Lower blood glucose reaction than sugar.
Hydrogenated starch hydrolysates	3	25-50	Does not cause cavities. Lower blood glucose reaction than sugar.

* % compared to sucrose

Foods containing nutritive sugar substitutes include gum, candies, chocolate, jams, ice cream, syrups and cough drops.

In the preceding chart, sugars with the suffix " ol " are also called *sugar alcohols* or *polyols*. They contain calories or carbohydrates and cause glucose levels in the blood to rise, but to a lesser degree than sugar. Effectively, these sugar alcohols are digested more slowly or are only partly absorbed in the intestine. As a result, blood glucose increases after their consumption, but only slightly.

9. Which non-nutritive sugar substitutes are found in foods?

The following chart lists the different non-nutritive sugar substitutes and their properties.

Non-nutritive sugar substitutes	Commercial names and/or foods that contain them	Sweetening power (%)*	ADI** mg/kg/ day	Comments
Acesulfame-potassium (K)	Carbonated drinks, puddings, gelatin, etc.	200	15	Does not cause cavities. Relatively stable under heat.
Aspartame	Packets of Equal® and blue packets of Sugar Twin®, puddings, gelatin, carbonated drinks, candies, etc.	160-220	40	Does not cause cavities. Composed of phenylalanine. Unstable under heat. Stability under heat increases when in capsule form.
Cyclamates	Packets of Sugar Twin® and Sucaryl®	30-80	11	Stable under heat.
Saccharin	Hermesetas®, Sweet'n Low®	200-700	5	Does not cause cavities.
Sucralose	Splenda® (Source® yogurt, etc.)	600	9	Does not cause cavities. Stable under heat.

* % compared to sugar. ** Acceptable daily intake.

10. **How are sugar alcohols listed in the facts nutrition chart of prepackaged foods?**

They are listed below total carbohydrates and are often mentioned by specific names or as sugar alcohols.

11. **In a product containing sugar alcohols, how do we measure the carbohydrate content that may affect blood glucose?**

There is an extract from a particular food product's nutritional chart, providing in this case information on carbohydrates:

Carbohydrates	19 g
Sugars	3 g
Sorbitol	16 g

For practical purposes, one rule applies to all sugar alcohols, despite the notable differences that exist between them. The grams of carbohydrates provided by a sugar alcohol are divided by two. This rule is based on the principle that these sugars are not completely digested.

For example: 16 g of sorbitol ÷ 2 = 8 g of carbohydrates absorbed

Of the 19 g of total carbohydrates in this food serving, 8 g of sorbitol will not be absorbed. As a result, no more than 11 g of carbohydrates can affect blood glucose levels (19 g of total carbohydrates – 8 g of sorbitol = 11 g of carbohydrates).

CHAPTER 10

Preparing a Menu

1. What steps should I follow when preparing a menu?

Example: spaghetti with meat sauce.

Step 1

➤ Refer to your **meal plan**.

➤ In your sample menu, find the number of recommended servings of each food group for the appropriate meal.

Example:

SAMPLE MENU	
Lunch	
Starches	3 servings
Fruit	1 serving
Vegetables	2 servings
Milk	1 serving
Meat/Meat substitutes	3 servings
Fat	1 serving

Step 2

➤   Assign the foods chosen to the proper group.

Spaghetti with meat sauce:

   spaghetti = the starch group;

   tomato and meat sauce = meat/meat substitutes and vegetable groups.

Step 3

➤   Find the serving size for each food chosen.

Starch
1 serving = 15 g carbohydrates

Food:	1 serving:
Spaghetti (cooked)	**125 ml (^{1}/2 cup)**

Meat and meat
substitutes

Food:	1 serving:
Lean ground beef	**30 g (1 oz.)**

Step 4

➤   Decide on the number of servings to be eaten. Example:

125 ml (^{1}/2 cup) of spaghetti	=	1 serving
therefore		
375 ml (1^1/2 cups)	=	3 servings
Tomato and meat sauce containing 90 g (3 oz.) of meat	=	3 servings of meat or meat substitutes and 1 serving of vegetables

In this case, the required servings of starch, meat and meat substitutes, along with one serving of vegetables, have been selected. The meal menu must then be completed with the other food groups (one serving of milk, one serving of vegetables, one serving of fruit and one serving of fat).

2. How can I figure out the nutritional value of a single serving?

To figure out the nutritional value of a single serving*, the following must be indicated:

1) the number of 15-g servings yielded per food item;

2) the nutritional value, given in grams (g), of the carbohydrates, proteins and fat provided by one serving or unit of this item.

Example:

PRUNE MUFFINS	
Ingredients:	flour, prunes, sugar, oil, eggs, baking soda
Servings or units:	18 muffins
Nutritional value per muffin:	28 g of carbohydrates, 5 g of fat

3. How can the nutritional value of a food portion be adapted to my meal plan?

If the meal plan is divided into 15-g servings of carbohydrates, you should determine how many servings of carbohydrates there are in all. Let's try this based on the muffin example above:

$$28 \text{ g} \div 15 \text{ g} = 1.9 = 2 \text{ servings of } 15 \text{ g}$$

It is important that you get to know your meal plan well, in order to be able to identify the foods you eat and place them in the appropriate food groups.

In this example, the prune muffin can be counted as one serving of fruit containing 15 g of carbohydrates and one serving of starch containing 15 g of carbohydrates.

---

* It is important to note that one serving of a particular recipe does not necessarily correspond to one serving of a particular food group (e.g., 1 muffin equals 1 individual recipe serving, but contains two 15-g servings of carbohydrates, that is, 30 g of carbohydrates per muffin).

The prune muffin also contains 5 g of fat. Since foods from the starch or fruit groups are not sources of fat, this muffin also provides one serving of fat, which must be accounted for in your daily food record.

The muffin can be adapted to the number of servings in a meal found in your sample menus.

For example:

SAMPLE MENU	
Lunch	
Starches	3 servings
Fruit	1 serving
Vegetables	2 servings
Milk	1 serving
Meat/Meat substitutes	3 servings
Fat	1 serving

In our example, one muffin counts as one serving of fruit, one serving of starch and one serving of fat. You will have to complete the meal with one serving of milk, two additional servings of starch, three servings of meat or meat substitutes, and two servings of vegetables.

If the meal plan is divided into fixed amounts of carbohydrates per meal, keep track of the carbohydrate content of the muffin or muffins that you eat. Complete the menu with the goal of reaching the recommended carbohydrate content for that particular meal.

4. How can we find out about the carbohydrate content of a food item if the yield per serving and the nutritional value are unknown?

If you do not know the nutritional value of a food item, it can be calculated from the list of ingredients, using a food composition table. For carbohydrate content, divide the total number of carbohydrates by the number of servings (or units) in the recipe.

CHAPTER 11

Special Situations

Eating Out

1. Can a person with diabetes eat out in a restaurant?

Yes. Occasional outings to restaurants are one of life's pleasures, and they need not be avoided because of diabetes. In order to enjoy the experience of eating out, the diner simply must come up with some good strategies allowing him or her to stick to the meal plan.

Even if restaurant meals are a daily ritual – pratised, for instance, every lunchtime – it is still possible to manage blood glucose levels. It is just simply a matter of choosing the right foods and the proper amounts. Nonetheless, we need to be wary of the fact that restaurant meals are on average 20% to 25% higher in fat than those prepared at home, and thus can lack nutritional balance. Furthermore, restaurant meals are also generally higher in sodium (salt) than home cooking. These factors pose a great challenge and must be taken into account.

2. What strategies can be helpful when choosing items from a restaurant menu?

Several strategies may prove helpful in choosing a meal from a restaurant menu.

1) Know your meal plan.

2) Ask about the ingredients that go into various menu items.

3)   Before you order, decide which food containing carbohydrates you want to eat. Combine it with a simple dish such as grilled meat rather than a mixed dish. This strategy will make it easier to adapt the menu to the food groups in your meal plan.

4)   Pay particular attention to food amounts.

5)   Choose a cooking method that uses a minimum of fat, such as grilling (meat) or poaching (fish).

6)   Do not eat the skin on barbecued chicken.

7)   Ask for sauces and salad dressings on the side whenever possible.

8)   Share French fries, pizza, cake or other such foods with a friend.

9)   Choose half servings or dishes from the children's menu.

10)   Order two entrees rather than an entree and a main course.

By getting into the habit of measuring and weighing servings of food, you will soon discover that your awareness of these portions will be quite keen. Many people find that, eventually, by trial and error, they are able to visually estimate the carbohydrate content of foods on the restaurant table. An easy method for determining meal portions is to use your hands as a measure. For more information, speak to a dietician.

Delayed Meals

1.   What effect does a delayed meal have on blood glucose levels?

A delayed meal may lead to hypoglycemia when the person with diabetes injects insulin or takes medications that stimulate the production of insulin by the pancreas (e.g., glyburide, gliclazide, repaglinide).

1)   If the meal is delayed about one hour:

Have a snack providing 15 g of carbohydrates at the scheduled mealtime and subtract this amount from the usual carbohydrate content of the meal.

2)   If the meal is delayed two to three hours:

Have the equivalent of one or two servings of starches (15 g to 30 g of carbohydrates) with a small amount of protein. Then, subtract these servings from the next meal or, if it happens to be the evening meal, simply replace the meal that was delayed with your evening snack.

> In each case, take oral antidiabetic medications or insulin with the delayed meal.

Alcohol

1.   Can a person with diabetes drink alcohol?

Alcohol may be consumed if the diabetes is well controlled. However, always remember that excessive alcohol intake can affect blood glucose levels, and may increase:

1)   blood pressure;

2)   triglycerides;

3)   body weight.

2.   What effect does alcohol have on blood glucose?

There are two types of alcoholic beverages:

1)   **alcoholic beverages that contain sugar**, such as beer, aperitif and sweet wines, these can raise blood glucose.

2)   **alcoholic beverages that do not contain sugar**; these comprise dry wines and distilled alcohols such as gin, rye, rum, whisky, vodka, cognac, armagnac etc., and do not raise blood glucose if they are consumed in small quantities.

People with diabetes that drink alcohol on an empty stomach may suffer from hypoglycemia, especially if they inject insulin or take medications that cause the pancreas to produce and release insulin (e.g., glyburide, gliclazide, repaglinide).

All alcoholic beverages can trigger **late hypoglycemia**. If alcohol is consumed with the evening meal, it may produce nocturnal hypoglycemia.

To avoid this risk:

1) have a snack before bed;

2) check blood glucose during the night, if advised to do so.

3. What factors should be considered when drinking alcohol?

1) Alcohol has a **high energy (caloric) value**. Its regular consumption may hinder weight loss and even cause weight gain if the calories in the alcohol are added to those calories in the meal plan.

2) Alcohol does not belong **to any food group in your meal plan**. Excessive consumption may be harmful to your health, especially if certain highly nutritious foods are left out of the regular food plan.

3) Excessive alcohol consumption may increase your **triglyceride levels** (a type of fat level in the blood) and **blood pressure**.

4. What guidelines can help a person with diabetes drink alcohol safely?

1) Only drink alcohol if the diabetes is well controlled.

2) Drink it with food — never on an empty stomach.

3) Consume alcohol in moderation:

➤ women should have no more than one drink a day (and more than nine per week);

➤ men should have no more than two drinks a day (and no more than 14 per week).

4) Drink it slowly.

5) Avoid consuming alcohol before, during or after physical activity.

> **One drink is:**
>
> $1^1/_2$ oz. (45 ml) of distilled alcohol
>
> 5 oz. (150 ml) of dry red or white wine
>
> 2 oz. (60 ml) of dry sherry
>
> 12 oz. (340 ml) of beer

Remember:

➤ Just one drink can lead to hypoglycemia.

➤ Just one drink can make your breath smell of alcohol ("fruity breath").

➤ Since the symptoms of hypoglycemia and drunkenness are very similar, people around you may confuse the two and delay appropriate treatment. Wear a bracelet or pendant that identifies you as a person with diabetes to make sure this does not happen.

5. What are the energy and carbohydrate values of alcoholic beverages?

The energy and carbohydrate values of various alcoholic beverages are shown in the following table.

Alcoholic beverages	Amount	Energy (calories)	Carbohydrates (grams)
Regular beer	340 ml (12 oz.)	150	13
Light beer	340 ml (12 oz.)	95	4
Beer with 0.5% alcohol / vol.	340 ml (12 oz.)	60 to 85	12 to 18
Low-carbohydrate beer	340 ml (12 oz.)	90	2.5
Wine coolers	340 ml (12 oz.)	170	22
Vodka Ice ®, Tornade ®	341 ml (12 oz.)	260	50
Sweet sherry	60 ml (2 oz.)	79	4
Sweet vermouth	60 ml (2 oz.)	96	10
Scotch	45 ml (1^1/2 oz.)	98	0
Rum	45 ml (1^1/2 oz.)	98	0
Dry white wine	150 ml (5 oz.)	106	1
Dry red wine	150 ml (5 oz.)	106	2
Champagne	150 ml (5 oz.)	120	2.5
Port	60 ml (2 oz.)	91	7
Crème de menthe	45 ml (1^1/2 oz.)	143	21
Coffee liqueur	45 ml (1^1/2 oz.)	159	17
Cognac	45 ml (1^1/2 oz.)	112	0

6. What can we use to replace alcoholic beverages?

Alcoholic beverages can be replaced with:

➤ low-sodium carbonated water;

➤ diet soft drinks;

➤ tomato juice with lemon or tabasco sauce;

➤ water with lemon and ice.

Minor Illnesses

1.   What effects do minor illnesses have on diabetes?

When people have diabetes, minor illnesses such as a cold, the flu or gastroenteritis can destabilize their blood sugar levels. Illnesses put stress on the body, and blood glucose levels tend to increase for two reasons:

➤ an increase in the secretion of certain hormones causes glucose stored in the liver to enter the bloodstream;

➤ these hormones also increase resistance to insulin, which hinders glucose from entering the cells.

These two reactions may therefore cause hyperglycemia.

2.   As a person with diabetes what precautions should I take when come down with a minor illness?

In the event of a minor illness, such as a cold or flu, that does not require medical attention, observe the five important rules that follow:

1)   Continue taking oral antidiabetic medications or insulin.

During illness, your insulin needs may increase. A person receiving insulin treatment may ask his or her physician for a sliding scale for insulin adjustment, according to blood glucose readings. For example, your doctor may prescribe the following:

Add one unit of rapid-acting insulin (Humalog® or NovoRapid®) or short-acting insulin (Humulin® R or Novolin® ge Toronto) for every mmol/l above 14 mmol/l before each meal and at bedtime, and during the night, if required.

2) Check your blood glucose levels at least four times a day or every two hours if you notice that they are high.

3) Check for ketone bodies in your urine or your blood when your blood glucose level is higher than 14 mmol/l.

4) Drink a lot of water to avoid dehydration.

5) Consume the recommended amount of carbohydrates for meals and snacks by eating foods that are easily digested.

3. Should the same precautions be taken for gastroenteritis?

Gastroenteritis generally causes diarrhea and may cause vomiting, which may lead to dehydration and the loss of electrolytes such as sodium and potassium, because of the inability to eat or drink.

Important!!!

Warn your doctor or go to the emergency department if one of the following situations occurs:

1) your blood glucose level rises above 20 mmol/l;

2) you observe the presence of ketone bodies (moderate or high levels) in your urine or blood;

3) you are vomiting and are unable to hold down liquids;

4) you have a fever with a temperature above 38.5°C (101.3°F) for more than 48 hours.

A three-phase approach is recommended to avoid dehydration and to reduce diarrhea and vomiting.

Phase 1: liquid food for the first 24 hours

Only consume liquids. Drink as much water, bouillon or consommé as you like. Drink liquids containing about 15 g of carbohydrates every hour. It may be preferable to drink 15 ml (1 tbs.) of these liquids every 15 minutes rather than every hour if larger amounts of liquid cannot be tolerated at once.

Oral rehydrating solutions such as Gastrolyte® and Pedialyte® are commercially available and may be a good alternative to the method described above. In addition, you might want to try a home remedy which consists of 250 ml (1 cup) of orange juice, the same amount of water and 2 ml (¹/2 tps.) of salt (250 ml or 1 cup of this drink equals 15 g of carbohydrate).

Over time, replace these drinks with juices, flavoured gelatin, regular decaffeinated and decarbonated soft drinks and nutritive supplements (e.g., Glucerna®, Resource® diabetic, etc.).

Phase 2: low residue foods (that do not tax the large intestine)

Gradually add solid foods containing 15 g of carbohydrates in order to reach the recommended carbohydrate content of the meal plan. For example:

- ➤ **fruits:** 1 small raw apple, grated, half a ripe banana, 125 ml (¹/2 cup) of unsweetened orange juice, etc.;

- ➤ **starches:** 2 rusks, 8 soda crackers, 4 Melba toasts, 1 toast, 125 ml (¹/2 cup) of plain pasta or 75 ml (¹/3 cup) of rice, etc.;

- ➤ **vegetables:** carrots, beets, asparagus, yellow or green beans, etc.;

- ➤ **meat:** lean meat such as white chicken or turkey, fish cooked without fat, mild cheese, etc.

Phase 3: Return to normal food

Gradually resume your normal diet according to the meal plan, while limiting the intake of:

➤ foods that may cause flatulence, such as corn, legumes (chickpeas, red beans, etc.), cabbage, onions, garlic and raw vegetables;

➤ foods that may cause irritation such as fried foods, spices, chocolate, coffee and cola.

Planning a Trip

1.   How should I plan a trip?

Because of your diabetes, you should take the following precautions when preparing a trip:

1) make sure your diabetes is **well controlled**;

2) obtain a **doctor's letter stating** that you have diabetes and describing your treatment, especially if you need insulin injections;

3) carry a **piece of identification** or bracelet indicating that you have diabetes;

4) find out what costs related to pre-existing illnesses are covered by **insurance companies** and if travel costs are included in the coverage, so you can get home in case of a medical emergency;

5) find out about the **customs and traditions** of the country you are visiting;

6) **inform the transportation company** that you have diabetes;

7) ask about required vaccines or other treatments (e.g., malaria prevention) at **travelers' clinic** or your doctor's office;

8)   prepare a **first-aid kit** including medication for diarrhea, vomiting and travel sickness; antibiotics may be included on the advice of your doctor;

9)   bring at least two pairs of **comfortable shoes**;

10) **avoid travelling alone.**

2.   What precautions should be taken when travelling with materials and medications necessary for the treatment of diabetes?

It is important to keep everything you need to treat your diabetes in your carry-on bag (and not luggage that will be stored separately), in particular:

1)   all medications with an identifying pharmacy label;

2)   twice the normal amount of insulin required for the trip, in case of breakage or in case the product is not available abroad. In some countries, insulin is packaged and sold in different concentrations (40 units/ml). Make sure, when injecting the insulin, that the syringe contains to the concentration normally used;

3)   an insulation storage container to protect insulin;

4)   extra syringes, even if a pen injector is used;

5)   a self-monitoring kit (glucose meter, test strips, etc.);

6)   food provisions in case of hypoglycemia or a delayed meal (e.g., dried or fresh fruit, juice, nuts, packets of peanut butter or cheese and crackers).

3.   What special recommendations should be followed during a trip?

Since you have diabetes, during a trip, you should follow the recommendations below:

1)   Follow your regular meal and snack schedule as closely as possible.

2)   Continue to check your blood glucose levels regularly to make sure your diabetes is always well controlled, since there is a good chance that you will have to change your routine.

3)   Always keep food provisions at hand in case of hypoglycemia or a delayed meal (e.g., dried or fresh fruit, juice, nuts, packets of peanut butter or cheese and crackers).

4)   Check your feet daily to rapidly identify any wounds.

4.   When treating diabetes with a "split-mixed" insulin regimen, how should the insulin doses be adjusted during a time-zone change of more than three hours?

The "split-mixed" insulin regimen is a combination of **intermediate-acting** NPH (Humulin® N or Novolin® ge) and one of two kinds of insulin: rapid-acting (Humalog® or NovoRapid®) or short-acting insulin (Humulin® R or Novolin® ge Toronto). The split-mixed regimen is injected before the morning and evening meals. Time zone changes can complicate the matter of when to take this medication.

Consider, for examples, a round trip between Montreal and Paris, which involves a the time-zone difference of six hours. Suppose you are taking the following insulin doses:

➤   Novolin® ge NPH 16 units and NovoRapid® (NR) 8 units before breakfast;

➤   Novolin® ge NPH 6 units and NovoRapid® (NR) 6 units before the dinner.

Departure:

Montreal–Paris. Since you lose six hours travelling to Paris, thus making your departure day six hours shorter, **reduce the NPH dose by 50% before the dinner.** In addition, eat only **half of the carbohydrates of your dinner before leaving, and the other half during the flight.** Consequently take **50% of the NR dose before dinner in Montreal and 50% before the evening in-flight meal.**

Meals	Blood glucose monitoring	Insulin	Meals
Montreal: breakfast	yes	NPH 16 units NR 8 units	normal
Montreal: lunch	yes	—	normal
Montreal: dinner	yes	NPH 3 units NR 3 units	50%
During flight: evening meal	yes	NR 3 units	50%
During flight: breakfast	yes	NPH 16 units NR 8 units	normal

Return:

Paris-Montreal. Since the return day is six hours longer than usual, you should take your **dinner during the flight** with the regular amount of NR insulin. Also, **have an additional dinner** equivalent to 50% of the carbohydrates of the regular dinner, **preceded by a dose of NR equal to 50% of the dose usually taken before the evening meal.** It is also recommended to delay the NPH dose until it is time for your extra evening meal.

Meals	Blood glucose monitoring	Insulin	Meals
Paris: breakfast	yes	NPH 16 units NR 8 units	normal normal
Paris: lunch	yes	—	normal
During flight: dinner	yes	NR 6 units	normal
Montreal: evening meal	yes	NPH 6 units NR 3 units	50%

5. **When treating diabetes with the multiple daily injections ("MDI") regimen with fixed carbohydrates, how should the insulin doses be adjusted during a time-zone change of more than three hours?**

The "MDI" regimen consists of one injection of rapid-acting (Humalog ® or NovoRapid ®) or short-acting (Humulin ® R or Novolin ® ge Toronto) insulin before each meal and one intermediate-acting (Humulin ® N or Novolin ® ge NPH) or long-acting (Humulin ® U or Lantus ®) insulin at bedtime.

Take as an example a round trip between Montreal and Paris, which involves a time-zone change of six hours. Suppose you take:

➤ NovoRapid ® (NR) 8 units before breakfast;

➤ NovoRapid ® (NR) 8 units before lunch;

➤ NovoRapid ® (NR) 8 units before the evening meal;

➤ Novolin ® ge NPH 8 units before bedtime.

Departure:

Montreal-Paris. The departure day being six hours shorter than usual, **take the NPH dose before dinner and take only 50% of it. Take half of the carbohydrates for dinner before take-off and the other half during the in-flight evening meal.** Also, take **50% of the NR dose before the dinner in Montreal and 50% before the evening meal during the flight.**

Meals	Blood glucose monitoring	Insulin	Meals
Montreal: breakfast	yes	NR 8 units	normal
Montreal: lunch	yes	NR 8 units	normal
Montreal: dinner	yes	NPH 4 units	
		NR 4 units	50%
During flight: evening meal	yes	NR 4 units	50%
During flight: breakfast	yes	NR 8 units	normal

Return:

Paris-Montreal. Having gained six hours on the final day of your trip — your return day being longer than usual — , **take the dinner** during the flight with the regular amount of NR insulin. It is further more advised to eat **an additional evening meal** containing 50% of the usual dinner's carbohydrates, **preceded by 50% of the NR dose usually taken before the first dinner.** Don't forget to delay the NPH dose until bedtime.

Meals	Blood glucose monitoring	Insulin	Meals
Paris: breakfast	yes	NR 8 units	normal
Paris: lunch	yes	NR 8 units	normal
During flight: dinner	yes	NR 8 units	normal
Montreal: evening meal	yes	NR 4 units	50%
Montreal: bedtime snack	yes	NPH 8 units	snack

6. When treating diabetes with the multiple daily injections ("MDI") insulin regimen with variable carbohydrates, how should insulin doses be adjusted during a trip with a time-zone change of over three hours?

The "MDI" insulin regimen with variable carbohydrates consists of one injection of rapid-acting (Humalog® or NovoRapid®) or short-acting (Humulin® R or Novolin® ge Toronto) insulin before each meal and one intermediate-acting (Humulin® N or Novolin® ge NPH) or long-acting (Humulin® U or Lantus®) insulin at bedtime.

Consider for example, a Montreal-Paris trip with a time-zone change of six hours. Suppose you usually take:

➤ Humalog® (Hg) 1.2 units/10 g of carbohydrates before breakfast;

➤ Humalog® (Hg) 1.0 unit/10 g of carbohydrates before lunch;

➨   Humalog® (Hg) 1.0 unit/10 g of carbohydrates before dinner;

➨   Humulin® U (UL) 12 units at bedtime.

Because of the longer duration of long-acting (UL) insulin, it is not necessary to change the dose.

Departure:

Montreal-Paris. In order to adjust to the fact that your day of departure is six hours shorter than usual, **move up the UL dose to** the appropriate time before take-off. While it is possible to wait until you are on the plane for your dinner, it is advisable to **have a light meal before leaving, along with Hg insulin** according to carbohydrate content. You may also take **an evening meal during the flight,** along with the same dose of Hg insulin per 10 g of carbohydrate as for dinner. **The next morning, during the flight, take Hg insulin before breakfast as usual.**

Meals	Blood glucose monitoring	Insulin	Meals
Montreal: breakfast	yes	Hg 1.2 units/10 g of carbohydrates	normal
Montreal: lunch	yes	Hg 1.0 unit/10 g of carbohydrates	normal
Montreal: dinner	yes	UL 12 units; Hg 1.0 unit/10 g of carbohydrates	50%
During flight: evening meal	yes	Hg 1.0 unit/10 g of carbohydrates	normal or 50%
During flight: breakfast	yes	Hg 1.2 units/10 g of carbohydrates	normal

Return:

Paris-Montreal. The return day being six hours longer, **take the dinner during the flight with the same dose of Hg insulin, and take an additional evening meal at night with the usual dose of Hg as for dinner. Take the UL at bedtime as usual.**

Meals	Blood glucose monitoring	Insulin	Meals
Paris: breakfast	yes	Hg 1.2 units/10 g of carbohydrates	normal
Paris: lunch	yes	Hg 1.0 unit/10 g of carbohydrates	normal
During flight: dinner	yes	Hg 1.0 unit/10 g of carbohydrates	normal
Montreal: evening meal	yes	Hg 1.0 unit/10 g of carbohydrates	normal or 50%
Montreal: bedtime snack	yes	UL 12 units	snack

7. When treating diabetes with the "premixed" insulin regimen, how should the insulin doses be adjusted during a trip involving a time-zone change of more than three hours?

The "premixed" insulin regimen consists of taking one injection containing a mix of rapid-acting or short-acting insulin and intermediate-acting insulin (Humulin® 30/70, Novolin® ge 30/70, Novolin® ge 50/50, Humalog® Mix 25, etc.) before breakfast and dinner.

Say, for example, that you go on a round trip between Montreal and Paris, which entails a time-zone change of six hours. Suppose you usually take Humulin® (H) 30/70 as follows:

➤ 20 units before breakfast;

➤ 10 units before dinner.

Departure:

Montreal-Paris. The departure day being six hours shorter than usual, **take half of the carbohydrates normally contained in the dinner before leaving and the other half during the flight. Also, take half the insulin dose with dinner before take-off, and the other half before the in-flight evening meal.**

Meals	Blood glucose monitoring	Insulin	Meals
Montreal: breakfast	yes	H 30/70 - 20 units	normal
Montreal: lunch	yes	—	normal
Montreal: dinner	yes	H 30/70 - 5 units	50%
During flight: evening meal	yes	H 30/70 - 5 units	50%
During flight: breakfast	yes	H 30/70 - 20 units	normal

Return:

Paris-Montreal. The return day being six hours longer, than usual **take an additional evening meal** (50% of the usual carbohydrate content) **preceded by a dose of insulin. This dose should be equivalent to 50% of the usual dose taken before dinner.**

Meals	Blood glucose monitoring	Insulin	Meals
Paris: breakfast	yes	H 30/70 - 20 units	normal
Paris: lunch	yes	—	normal
During flight: dinner	yes	H 30/70 - 10 units	normal
Montreal: evening meal	yes	H 30/70 - 5 units	50%
Montreal: bedtime snack	yes	—	snack

CHAPTER 12

Oral Antidiabetic Medications

1. What is oral antidiabetic medication?

It is medication **taken orally** that **lowers blood glucose levels**.

2. In what situations and under what circumstances should oral antidiabetic medications be used in the treatment of diabetes?

Oral antidiabetic medications are used to treat type 2 diabetes **if diet, exercise and weight loss programs are not sufficient to normalize blood glucose levels**. They can be taken alone or in combination.

> WARNING: Oral antidiabetic medications do not replace, but rather complement, diet, exercise and weight loss programs.

3. How many classes of oral antidiabetic medications are there?

There are six classes of oral antidiabetic medications, as illustrated in this table:

Classes	Medications
Sulfonylureas*	Chlorpropamide (e.g., Apo®-Chlorpropamide) Gliclazide (e.g., Diamicron®) Glimepiride (Amaryl®) Glyburide (e.g., Diaβeta®, Euglucon®) Tolbutamide (e.g., Apo®-Tolbutamide)
Amino acid derivatives*	Nateglinide (Starlix®)
Meglitinides*	Repaglinide (GlucoNorm®)
Biguanides	Metformin (e.g., Glucophage®)
Thiazolidinediones	Pioglitazone (Actos®) Rosiglitazone (Avandia®)
Alpha-glucosidase inhibitors	Acarbose (Prandase®)

* Insulin secretagogues

4. What are the characteristics of sulfonylureas (e.g., Diaβeta®, Diamicron®, Amaryl®)?

1) **Mechanism of action:** Sulfonylureas **stimulate the pancreas to produce more insulin** (they are known as insulin secretagogues). They are therefore ineffective if the insulin-producing cells of the pancreas no longer function.

2) **Adverse effects: Hypoglycemia** is the most common side effect attributed to sulfonylureas. It may occur at any time of day or night; therefore, dosage should be adjusted accordingly. In order to minimize the risk of hypoglycemia, meals and snacks should be eaten at regular hours as scheduled in the meal plan. These medications should not be taken at bedtime.

3) **When to take them:** It is advisable to take sulfonylureas **before meals, but never more than 30 minutes before them**. Sulfonylureas such as modified release gliclazide (Diamicron® MR) and glimepiride (Amaryl®), should be taken once a day with breakfast.

5. What are the characteristics of nateglinide (Starlix®) and repaglinide (GlucoNorm®)?

1) **Mechanism of action:** Like sulfonylureas, nateglinide and repaglinide stimulate **the pancreas to produce more insulin** (they also are insulin secretagogues). Therefore, they too are ineffective if the insulin-producing cells of the pancreas no longer function. They act faster and for a shorter period than sulfonylureas.

2) **Adverse effects: Hypoglycemia** is the side effect most commonly attributed to nateglinide and repaglinide. Dosage should be adjusted accordingly. In order to minimize the risk of hypoglycemia, meals and snacks should be taken at regular hours, as scheduled in the meal plan. These medications should not be taken at bedtime.

3) **When to take them:** These medications should be taken **as close as possible to the beginning of a meal (0 to 15 minutes) but no more than 30 minutes before it.**

6. What are the characteristics of metformin (e.g., Glucophage®)?

1) **Mechanism of action:** Metformin **reduces the production of glucose** by the liver.

2) **Adverse effects: Intestinal problems, especially diarrhea,** are the side effects most commonly attributed to metformin. Some patients also note a slight metallic aftertaste. When taken on its own, metformin is rarely associated with hypoglycemia.

3) **When to take it:** Take metformin **at mealtime** in order to minimize adverse intestinal effects.

7. What are the characteristics of pioglitazone (Actos ®) and rosiglitazone (Avandia ®)?

1) **Mechanism of action:** Pioglitazone and rosiglitazone **lower insulin resistance**; in other words, they increase the effectiveness of insulin. These insulin sensitizing drugs help to achieve an increase in glucose use, especially by muscle tissue, but also adipose tissue.

2) **Adverse effects: Edema** (swelling due to water retention) and **weight gain** are possible side effects. When taken on their own, however, pioglitazone and rosiglitazone are rarely associated with hypoglycemia.

3) **When to take them:** These medications should always be taken at the same time of day, usually in the morning. It is not necessary to take them with meals.

8. What are the characteristics of acarbose (Prandase ®)?

1) **Mechanism of action:** Acarbose **slows the absorption of carbohydrates ingested during meals.** It also helps to control rising blood glucose levels after meals.

2) **Adverse effects: Digestive problems, especially bloating and flatulence,** are the side effects most commonly attributed to acarbose. Acarbose is not associated with hypoglycemia when take on its own.

3) **When to take it**: Acarbose should be taken **with the first mouthful** of your meal to ensure its effectiveness.

9. What should I do if I miss a dose of my oral antidiabetic medication?

1) If you notice the omission quickly, take the dose immediately. If not, skip the missed dose and wait for the next scheduled one.

2) **Never double the dose.**

3) It is not advisable to take sulfonylureas, nateglinide or repaglinide at bedtime, as this increases the risk of nocturnal hypoglycemia.

4) Acarbose is only effective when taken **with a meal**. If you forget to take it at mealtime, do not bother to take it afterwards.

10. Do oral antidiabetic medications interact with other medications?

All medications can potentially interact with other agents. Anticipating and preventing such interactions is the responsibility of pharmacists and doctors, but the patient also has a role to play in this regard.

All people taking medication should keep an up-to-date list of their prescriptions (e.g., in a self-monitoring logbook). You are strongly advised to **bring your medications in their containers with you** when seeing your doctor, to help him or her make the right decisions regarding your treatment. In addition, try to find a regular pharmacist, so that he or she can get to know you and your medical history. The pharmacist will then be able to detect and anticipate certain problems and give you proper advice.

11. Is it necessary to take oral antidiabetic medication all your life?

In general, oral antidiabetic medication must be taken over the long term, because, at this point in time, diabetes is a disease that can be controlled but not cured. Treatment must still be regularly adjusted (and doses either increased or decreased), by your doctor. The goal of medications is to normalize blood glucose levels so as to avoid unpleasant side effects such as hypoglycemia.

Medication	Glyburide	Gliclazide	Modified-release gliclazide	Glimepiride	Repaglinide
Class	Sulfonylureas (insulin secretagogues)	Sulfonylureas (insulin secretagogues)	Sulfonylureas (insulin secretagogues)	Sulfonylureas (insulin secretagogues)	Meglitinides (insulin secretagogues)
Commercial name (non-exhaustive list)	Diaßeta Euglucon Apo-Glyburide Gen-Glybe Novo-Glyburide	Diamicron Gen-Gliclazide Novo-Gliclazide	Diamicron MR	Amaryl	GlucoNorm
Common form	2.5 mg and 5 mg tablets (divisible in two)	80 mg tablets (divisible in four)	30 mg tablets (non-divisible)	1 mg, 2 mg and 4 mg tablets (divisible in two)	0.5 mg, 1 mg and 2 mg tablets (non-divisible)
Daily dosage	1.25 mg to 20 mg	40 mg to 320 mg	30 mg to 120 mg	1 mg to 8 mg	1 mg to 16 mg
Number of daily doses	1 to 3	1 to 3	1	1	2 to 4 (according to the number of meals)
When to take it	0 to 30 min before meal	0 to 30 min before meal	At breakfast	At breakfast	0 to 15 min before meal
Most common adverse effects	Hypoglycemia	Hypoglycemia	Hypoglycemia	Hypoglycemia	Hypoglycemia
Risk of hypoglycemia	Yes	Yes	Yes	Yes	Yes

Nateglinide	Acarbose	Metformin	Pioglitazone	Rosiglitazone	Rosiglitazone and metformin
Amino acid derivative (insulin secretagogues)	Alpha-glucosidases inhibitor	Biguanides	Thiazolidinediones	Thiazolidinediones	Thiazolidinediones and biguanides
Starlix	Prandase	Glucophage Apo-Metformin Gen-Metformin Novo-Metformin	Actos	Avandia	Avandamet
60 mg, 120 mg and 180 mg tablets (non-divisible)	50 mg and 100 mg tablets (divisible in two)	500 mg (divisible in two) and 850 mg tablets (non-divisible)	15 mg, 30 mg and 45 mg tablets (non-divisible)	2 mg, 4 mg and 8 mg tablets (non-divisible)	(rosiglitazone/metformin) 1 mg/500 mg, 2 mg/500 mg and 4 mg/500 mg tablets (non-divisible)
180 mg to 540 mg	50 mg to 300 mg	250 mg to 2,500 mg	15 mg to 45 mg	4 mg to 8 mg	2mg/1,000 mg to 8mg/2,000 mg
3	1 to 3	1 to 4	1	1 to 2	2
0 to 15 min before meal	First mouthful	At mealtime	With or without food	With or without food	At mealtime
Hypoglycemia	Bloating, flatulence, diarrhea	Diarrhea, metallic taste	Edema, weight gain	Edema, weight gain	Edema, weight gain, diarrhea, metallic taste
Yes	No	No	No	No	No

MECHANISMS OF ACTION OF ORAL ANTIDIABETIC MEDICATIONS

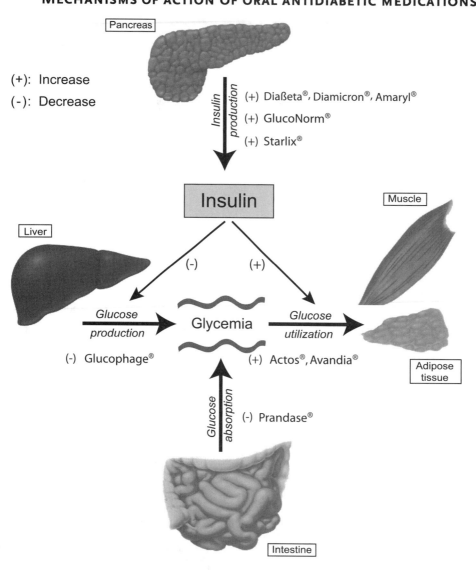

Pancreas

(+): Increase
(-): Decrease

Insulin production

(+) Diaßeta®, Diamicron®, Amaryl®

(+) GlucoNorm®

(+) Starlix®

Insulin

Muscle

Liver

(-)   (+)

Glucose production   Glycemia   *Glucose utilization*

(-) Glucophage®   (+) Actos®, Avandia®

Adipose tissue

Glucose absorption

(-) Prandase®

Intestine

- ➤ Diaßeta ®, Diamicron ®, Amaryl ®, GlucoNorm ®, and Starlix ® causes the pancreas to produce more insulin (the insulin secretagogues).

- ➤ Glucophage ® (metformin) decreases the production of glucose by the liver.

- ➤ Actos ® and Avandia ® stimulate insulin action that increases the use of glucose, especially by the muscles, but also by adipose (fatty) tissue.

- ➤ Prandase ® delays the absorption of dietary carbohydrates.

CHAPTER 13

Over-the-Counter Medications

1. What are over-the-counter medications?

Over-the-counter medications include all medication available without a prescription. Some may only be obtained after consulting your pharmacist, while others can be purchased on the spot.

2. When and how should over-the-counter medications be used?

Over-the-counter medications allow people to self-medicate **mild health problems**. They should only be used on a temporary basis, that is, for short periods of time, in order to prevent the drugs from masking the symptoms of a more serious condition. All directions and warnings printed on the product's packaging should be followed closely.

3. Are over-the-counter medications free of side effects?

No medication is completely free of side effects. In some cases, over-the-counter medications may cause harmful side effects. Some of these medications should be avoided or used with care in the case of certain illnesses. Furthermore interactions between over-the-counter and prescribed medications are not uncommon.

4.   How can I be sure to choose over-the-counter medications that are safe for me?

It is strongly recommended that you talk to your pharmacist before choosing an over-the-counter medication. The pharmacist can indicate the product most appropriate for your condition, by taking into consideration your symptoms, your health problems and any other medications you may be taking; he or she may even suggest certain non-pharmacological measures. The pharmacist will advise you to consult your doctor if he or she believes your condition requires it. Always have your prescriptions filled by the same pharmacist, who will therefore be familiar with your medical file and in a better position to give you advice.

5.   Which over-the-counter medications should be avoided or used cautionsly by people with diabetes?

The following medications should be used with caution:

1)   **oral decongestants** (for the treatment of nasal congestion);

2)   medications containing **sugar**;

3)   **keratolytic preparations** (for the treatment of corns, calluses and warts);

4)   high doses of **acetylsalicylic acid** (e.g., Aspirin® or ASA).

6.   Why must oral decongestants be used cautionsly?

Oral decongestants (e.g., Sudafed®) are medications (available in syrups, tablets or powders) that reduce nasal congestion. The majority of oral decongestants contain a "sympathomimetic" ingredient (e.g., pseudoephedrine) that can have a **hyperglycemic** effect, especially if recommended doses are exceeded; and these types of products are frequently overconsumed. Cold medications often contain a mixture of ingredients (to relieve coughs, fight fevers, etc.)that includes a sympathomimetic decongestant. It is not uncommon for people to take two different products when treating their colds or flus. By so doing, they unwittingly double the dosage of the decongestant.

Moveover, oral decongestants of this kind are further not recommended for people with vascular problems, hypertension, hyperthyroidism and cardiac diseases such as angina.

As an alternative, it is advisable to drink plenty of water, keep the room well humidified and use a saline nasal vaporizer. If the condition persists, use a nasal decongestant vaporizer, but for no longer than 72 hours (to avoid rebound congestion).

7. Why should medications containing sugar be used cautionsly?

It is important for people with diabetes to know which medications contain sugar in order to properly maintain, control, and manage blood glucose levels. Sugar is present not only in syrups, but also in powders, chewable tablets, lozenges, etc. A person with diabetes must avoid any medication which contains **20 calories** (5 g of carbohydrates) **per dose or providing more than 80 calories** (20 g of carbohydrates) **per day**. If you do take these medications on occasion, it is important to include them in the overall carbohydrate tally of your meal plan. The sugar content of medecinal products may be printed on their packaging; if not, your pharmacist can give you this information.

There are many "sucrose-free" or "sugar-free" preparations. These usually contain sugar substitutes and can be used by people with diabetes at the recommended dose, provided that the active ingredient is not contraindicated for another reason.

8. Why should keratolytic preparations (for the treatment of corns, calluses and warts) be used cautiously?

Adhesive plasters, pads, ointments or gels containing products such as acetylsalicylic or tannic acid are often used to treat corns, calluses and warts. These acids are **highly irritating**. See a doctor, a podiatrist or a nurse who is a specialist in foot care before using these products.

9.   Why should high doses of acetylsalicylic acid be used with caution?

High doses of acetylsalicylic acid (e.g., Aspirin®, ASA, Anacin®, Entrophen®, etc.) can cause hypoglycemia if the daily dose exceeds 4,000 mg— the equivalent of more than twelve 325 mg tablets per day or more than eight 500 mg tablets per day.

Acetaminophen (e.g., Tylenol®, Atasol®, etc.) does not contain acetylsalicylic acid and is a safe alternative for the treatment of fever and pain.

10.   Is there a simple way to find out which over-the-counter medications should be used cautionsly or even avoided? Is anything available at my local pharmacy?

In Quebec, the Ordre des pharmaciens du Québec has developed a program called the "code médicament" (or "Drug Caution Code"). This code consists of six letters, with each letter corresponding to a specific warning. These code letters usually appear on the price sticker or the particular shelf where the medication is placed.

The **code letter** *E* is specifically for people with diabetes. Products bearing a "code E" are **not recommended**. This code identifies three types of products:

1)   oral decongestants;

2)   medications with a sugar content equal to 20 calories or more **per dose** or 80 calories or more **per day**, according to the recommended dose;

3)   keratolytic preparations (for the treatment of corns, calluses and warts).

A personalized "code médicament" card filled out by your pharmacist will indicate the code letters that apply to you.

If you are not a Quebec resident, check with your pharmacist to find out if there is a similar program in your area.

11. Can "natural" products be used by people with diabetes?

Many "natural" products are commercially available. It is important to know that "natural" does not necessarily mean "innocuous". In fact, some natural products may have dangerous side effects or interact with prescribed medications. Others are contraindicated for various illnesses.

Furthermore, the quality of natural products can vary widely, and it is not always possible to know exactly what these products are made of.

If people with diabetes choose to use a natural product, they should talk to a pharmacist and have him or her verify that the product is suitable. Moreover doctors should be informed of the products used by their patients.

12. Can natural products have an effect on blood glucose levels?

Some natural products can raise blood glucose levels, while others can lower them. Glucosamine, a supplement used in the case of osteoarthritis, is an example of a product that may raise glucose levels. Fenugrec, vanadium, bitter melon (*Momordica charantia*) and Gymnema sylvestre are products that can lower them.

Consult your pharmacist or your doctor before consuming a natural product, to make sure it is both safe and effective. If you decide to take a potentially hyperglycemic or hypoglycemic product, be sure to check its effect on your blood glucose level.

Finally, according to currently available information and research, no natural product can be recommended as a replacement for oral antidiabetic medications or insulin.

CHAPTER 14

Insulins

1. What is the role of insulin?

Insulin is a hormone that plays an important role in maintaining normal blood glucose levels. It can be seen as a kind of glucose "manager," controlling glucose levels. Insulin allows blood glucose to enter the cells of the body and also affects the liver by lowering its production of glucose. These two actions help to lower blood glucose levels.

2. When is insulin indicated for the treatment of diabetes?

Insulin is systematically used to treat **type 1 diabetes** because, in this case, the pancreas produces no insulin. It can also be used for **type 2 diabetes** if diet, exercise, weight loss and oral antidiabetic medications **are not sufficient to control blood glucose levels.**

3. How are insulins produced?

Insulins are primarily manufactured in laboratories according to biogenetic techniques that use bacteria or yeast genetically programmed to produce insulin.

There are two categories of insulin:

1) **Human insulin:** This insulin is identical to the one produced by the pancreas. All insulins called Humulin® or Novolin® belong to this category.

2) Analogue insulin: This insulin is similar to the one produced by the pancreas. However, its structure has been slightly modified in comparison with that of human insulin in order to give it new properties. Humalog®, NovoRapid® and Lantus® are some examples.

Certain types of insulin may also be of animal origin (purified pork insulin). These types are seldom ever used. They are mentioned here for informational purposes only.

4.   What are the different types of insulin?

Insulin preparations can be classified according to their action time. The following terms will help us to differentiate the later:

➤   **onset of action:** the time insulin takes to start working;

➤   **peak of action:** the time during which the insulin is at maximum effectiveness;

➤   **duration of action:** the duration of the insulin's effectiveness in the body.

There are six types of insulin:

1)   rapid-acting insulin;

2)   short-acting insulin;

3)   intermediate-acting insulin;

4)   long-acting insulin;

5)   premixed insulins made of a mixture of **rapid-acting** and **intermediate-acting** insulins;

6)   premixed insulins made of a mixture of **short-acting** and **intermediate-acting** insulins.

5. What are the action times of the different types of insulin?

Type of insulin	Onset of action	Peak of action	Duration of action
Rapid-acting			
Humalog® (lispro)	0 to 15 minutes	1 to 2 hours	3 to 4 hours
NovoRapid® (aspart)	0 to 10 minutes	1 to 3 hours	3 to 5 hours
Short-acting			
Humulin® R (regular)	30 minutes	2 to 4 hours	6 to 8 hours
Novolin® ge Toronto			
Intermediate-acting			
Humulin® N	1 to 2 hours	6 to 12 hours	18 to 24 hours
Novolin® ge NPH			
Humulin® L			
Long-acting			
Humulin® U	4 to 5 hours	8 to 20 hours (small)	24 to 28 hours
Lantus® (glargine) [1]	1 hour	none	24 hours
Premixed rapid-acting and intermediate-acting			
Humalog® Mix 25 [2]	0 to 15 minutes	1 to 2 hours and 6 to 12 hours	18 to 24 hours
Premixed short-acting and intermediate-acting [3]			
Novolin® ge 10/90	30 minutes	2 to 4 hours and 6 to 12 hours	18 to 24 hours
Novolin® ge 20/80			
Humulin® 30/70			
Novolin® ge 30/70			
Novolin® ge 40/60			
Novolin® ge 50/50			

[1] Lantus® is a long-acting analogue insulin which should soon be available in Canada. Currently, it is used in certain special cases (e.g., for serious hypoglycemia).

[2] Humalog® Mix 25 is a mixture of 25% lispro insulin (rapid-acting insulin) and 75% lispro protamine insulin (intermediate-acting insulin).

[3] The first number corresponds to the percentage of short-acting insulin and the second, to the percentage of intermediate-acting NPH insulin.

OUTLINE OF VARIOUS TYPES OF INSULIN

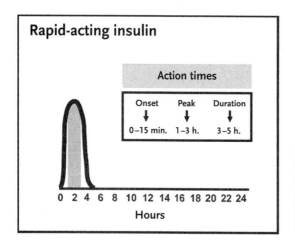

Rapid-acting insulin

Action times

Onset	Peak	Duration
0–15 min.	1–3 h.	3–5 h.

Hours

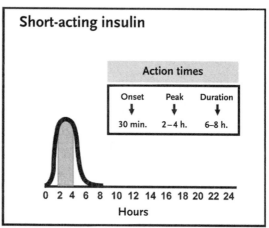

Short-acting insulin

Action times

Onset	Peak	Duration
30 min.	2–4 h.	6–8 h.

Hours

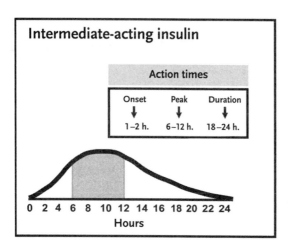

Intermediate-acting insulin

Action times

Onset	Peak	Duration
1–2 h.	6–12 h.	18–24 h.

Hours

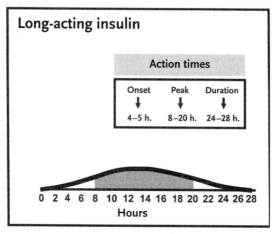

Long-acting insulin

Action times

Onset	Peak	Duration
4–5 h.	8–20 h.	24–28 h.

Hours

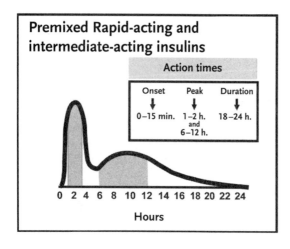

Premixed Rapid-acting and intermediate-acting insulins

Action times

Onset	Peak	Duration
0–15 min.	1–2 h. and 6–12 h.	18–24 h.

Hours

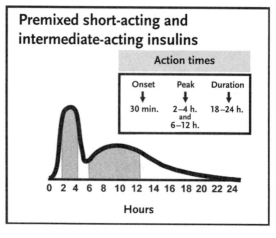

Premixed short-acting and intermediate-acting insulins

Action times

Onset	Peak	Duration
30 min.	2–4 h. and 6–12 h.	18–24 h.

Hours

6.   How many insulin injections are required per day?

In general, insulin treatment requires one, two, three or four injections a day. The daily number of injections, the types of insulin used and the timing of injections must be determined according to the condition of the person with diabetes. Treatment should also be adapted to the person's lifestyle. The goal is to maintain blood glucose levels as close to normal as possible.

7.   What are the most frequently prescribed insulin regimens?

There are several insulin regimens; here are four of the most commonly prescribed ones:

1)   The "**split-mixed**" regimen consists of injecting an intermediate-acting insulin and either a rapid-acting or a short-acting insulin before breakfast and dinner. The dinnertime injection of intermediate-acting insulin is sometimes given at bedtime in order to prevent nocturnal hypoglycemia.

2)   The "**multiple daily injections (MDI)**" regimen consists of injecting a rapid-acting or short-acting insulin before each meal and an intermediate-acting or long-acting basal insulin at bedtime. Although basal insulin is usually given in one injection, it can also be administered in several injections throughout the day, if so desired.

The rapid-acting or short-acting insulin dose may be fixed (fixed carbohydrate regimen) or calculated according to the amount of carbohydrates consumed in the meal (variable carbohydrate regimen). In a variable carbohydrate diet, the insulin dose is set by ratio, for example, 1 unit/10g of carbohydrates, that is, 1 unit of insulin per 10 g of carbohydrates consumed.

3)   The "**premixed**" regimen consists of injecting a mixed dose of either rapid-acting or short-acting insulin and intermediate-acting insulin before breakfast and dinner.

PRINCIPAL INSULIN REGIMENS

Split-mixed regimen

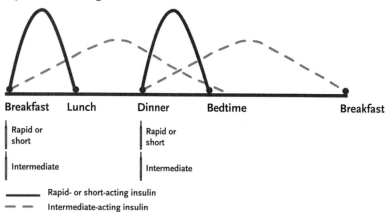

Multiple daily injection (MDI) regimen (with intermediate-acting insulin)

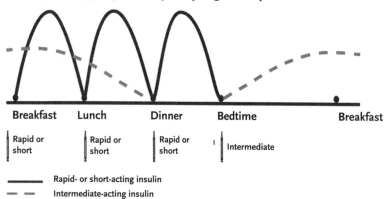

Multiple daily injection (MDI) regimen (with long-acting insulin)

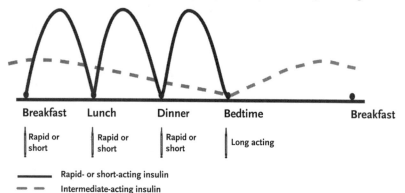

Pre-mixed regimen

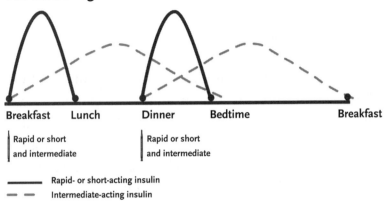

| Breakfast | Lunch | | Dinner | Bedtime | | Breakfast |

| Rapid or short and intermediate | | Rapid or short and intermediate |

———— Rapid- or short-acting insulin

— — Intermediate-acting insulin

Combined regimen

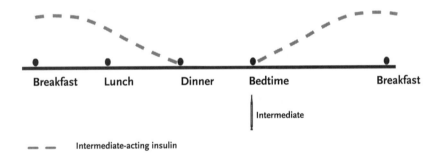

| Breakfast | Lunch | Dinner | Bedtime | | Breakfast |

Intermediate

— — Intermediate-acting insulin

4) The "**combined**" regimen consists of injecting intermediate-acting or long-acting insulin at bedtime, along with the usual oral antidiabetic medications that are taken during the day.

8. What is intensive insulinotherapy?

Intensive insulinotherapy consists of multiple insulin injections (e.g., the "multiple daily injections (MDI)" regimen) or the use of an insulin pump combined with blood glucose measurements, as well as insulin doses that must be self-adjusted by the person with diabetes. Intensive insulinotherapy is essentially an attempt to imitate the normal release of insulin by the pancreas. The goal of this treatment is to maintain blood glucose values as close to normal as possible.

9. What are the insulin doses required to control blood glucose?

Insulin doses are initially determined by your doctor and vary according to your blood glucose readings. The doses are measured in **units**. Some people inject themselves with fixed doses, while others set their doses in proportion to the carbohydrate content of their meals. Whatever the regimen used, insulin doses should be modified frequently according to various factors such as diet, exercise and periods of illness.

10. When should insulin be injected with respect to meals and to bedtime?

Meals:

➤ **Rapid-acting insulin** should be injected **just before meals** (or no more than 15 minutes before if Humalog® is used, and no more than 10 minutes before if NovoRapid® is used), whether the insulin is premixed or not.

➤ **Short-acting insulin** should be injected **15 to 30 minutes before meals**, whether it is premixed or not.

This allows for the peak action of the insulin to coincide with the peak absorption of the ingested carbohydrates.

Bedtime:

➡ **Intermediate-acting or long-acting insulin** is generally injected at about 10 p.m. Injection time must be as regular as possible.

This allows for the peak action to coincide with your breakfast meal (in the case of intermediate-acting insulin).

11. What is the most common adverse effect of insulin treatment?

Hypoglycemia is the most common adverse effect observed in people treated with insulin. The risk of hypoglycemia is much higher during the peak action of insulin, as this is the time when your insulin is working at its greatest effect. Sound knowledge about insulin and the rules governing its dosage adjustment will help you in lowering the risk of hypoglycemia.

12. How can diabetes be well controlled with insulin?

To control diabetes with insulin injections in the best possible way, it is important to:

1) follow your **meal plan** closely ;

2) **check your blood glucose levels regularly;**

3) **be well informed about the insulin you use;** and

4) **self-adjust your insulin doses** after receiving the necessary training from your diabetes care team.

13. When should a person with diabetes receiving insulin treatment check his or her blood glucose?

A person with diabetes on insulin treatment should take a blood glucose reading **before meals and at bedtime (before a snack)**. It may also be helpful to occasionally measure blood glucose after meals (one or two hours after the first mouthful). Readings can sometimes be taken during the night (at about 2 a.m.), for example, if you wake up feeling irritable or with a headache. On sick days, it is advisable to increase the frequency of blood glucose measurements. In addition, blood glucose should be checked every time a person with diabetes feels unwell, to see if this condition is due to hypoglycemia or hyperglycemia.

CHAPTER 15

Preparation and Injection of Insulin

1. What devices can be used for injecting insulin?

Two types of devices are commonly available for the injection of insulin.

1) **The Syringe:** It is a device consisting of a cylinder and a plunger that is fitted with a fine needle. Syringes come in sizes of either 100, 50, or 30 units capacity. It is important to note that the finer the needle, the greater the needle's gauge. A 30-gauge needle, for example, is finer than a 29-gauge needle. However, the finer the needle (and the larger its gauge), the shorter it is. For example, the 30-gauge needle is 8 mm long, while the 29-gange needle measures 12.7 mm).

2) **Pen injector:** Slightly larger than a pen, it is made up of three parts – the cap, which covers a fine needle, the cartridge holder, which contains the insulin cartridge, and the pen body, which includes the plunger. A dosage dial allows you to select the desired dose.

2. How do you prepare a syringe with a specific type of insulin?

There are three steps in the preparation and injection of a specific insulin with a syringe.

Preparing the materials

1) **Wash your hands** with soap and water and dry them well.

2) Lay out the **materials**: syringe, insulin vial, alcohol swab, and cotton ball.

   ➡ Use a new syringe for each injection.

   ➡ Use a vial of insulin that has been stored at room temperature.

3) Check the label on the vial to make sure you have the right **type of insulin**.

4) Check the **expiry dates** on the label, namely, the date printed by the manufacturer and the date you recorded on your vial after opening the bottle.

   ➡ It is recommended that you **use a 29-gauge syringe measuring 12.7 mm** when injecting **Humulin® U insulin**; this will make injections easier and prevent needle blockage.

Preparing the insulin

1) If the **insulin is cloudy**, you should roll the vial between your hands and turn it upside down, to ensure that the contents are mixed thoroughly and that the preparation is uniformly cloudy or milky (**do not shake the vial**).

2) **Disinfect the cap of the vial** with the alcohol swab.

3) **Pull back the plunger** of the syringe to draw in a volume of air equal to the amount of insulin to be injected.

4) **Insert the needle** in the rubber cap of the insulin vial.

5) **Push down the plunger in order to inject the air** into the vial.

6) **Turn the vial and syringe** upside down. Make sure the tip of the needle is still in the insulin.

7) **Pull the plunger back gently** in order to draw in the number of insulin units needed for the injection.

   ➡ Make sure there are no air bubbles in the syringe; if there are, you may in fact inject a smaller amount of insulin than is required.

   ➡ Push the plunger until air bubbles disappear.

➤ Check the syringe to make sure no insulin has been lost; if this has happened, draw more solution into the syringe.

Injecting insulin and recording the data

1) **Where to inject the insulin.**

    ➤ Avoid injecting insulin into a limb or part of the body that will be used for an upcoming physical activity (e.g., a leg, if you plan to take a walk or an arm, if you intend to play tennis, etc.).

2) **Choose the injection site** paying special attention to the condition of the skin.

    ➤ Avoid any depression, bump, growth, bruise, blotch or painful spot.

3) **Disinfect the skin** with an alcohol swab or with soap and water and let it dry.

    ➤ Make sure the injection site is clean. At home, it is not absolutely necessary to use alcohol to clean the site – this is optional.

4) **Pinch the skin between the thumb and forefinger and keep pinching it** until the end of the injection.

5) Hold the syringe like a pencil and **pierce the skin**.

    ➤ The insulin should be injected into subcutaneous tissue (the tissue beneath the skin).

6) **Inject all the insulin** by, pushing the plunger all the way down with a quick and smooth motion. You can now stop pinching your skin.

    ➤ **Do not pull the plunger back:** If you raise the plunger to check whether or not you hit the right spot, you may damage the skin.

    ➤ **Leave the needle in place** for about **five seconds**.

7) **Withdraw the needle** and delicately press a cotton ball onto the injection site.

8) **Record the number of insulin units** injected as well as the type of insulin used in the appropriate column of your self-monitoring logbook.

3. What precautions should be taken when mixing two types of insulin in the same syringe?

When mixing clear and cloudy insulin in the same syringe, certain precautions are necessary:

1) To make sure that the cloudy insulin does not enter the clear insulin bottle, it is important to mix the insulins properly. However, the preferred order of preparing the insulins varies somewhat among healthcare professionals. Most of these professionals recommend preparing the clear rapid-acting Humalog ® or NovoRapid ®) or short-acting (Humulin ® R or Novolin ® ge Toronto) insulin before the cloudy (Humulin ® N or Novolin ® ge NPH) insulin. **On the other hand, some of them suggest that you prepare cloudy insulin before the clear one, in order to easily detect any contamination of the clear insulin by the cloudy. Both options are acceptable.**

2) If one insulin is contaminated by the other, the contaminated vial must be discarded, because its time of action (start, peak, duration) may have been modified. An insulin contaminated by another one can hinder the control of blood glucose.

3) It is important to always prepare insulins in the same order so as to prevent errors in their preparation.

4) In general, you should not mix long-acting (Humulin ® U) insulin or intermediate-acting (Humulin ® L) insulin with either rapid-acting (Humalog ® or NovoRapid ®) or short-acting (Humulin ® R ou Novolin ® ge Toronto) insulin.

5) As a rule of thumb, only mix insulins from the same manufacturer in the same syringe.

6)   The Lantus ® (glargine) insulin available in some countries must never be mixed with another type of insulin.

4.   How do you prepare and inject two types of insulin with the same syringe?

There are three steps in the preparation and injection of two types of insulin with a single syringe.

Preparing the materials

1)   **Wash your hands** with soap and water and dry them well.

2)   Lay out the **materials**: Syringe, insulin vials, alcohol swab, cotton ball.

> Use a new syringe for each injection.

> Use vials of insulin stored at room temperature.

3)   Check the labels of the vials to make sure you have the right **types of insulin**.

4)   Check the **expiry dates** on the labels, specifically, the dates printed by the manufacturer and the dates you recorded after opening the vials.

> It is recommended that you **use a 29-gauge syringe measuring 12.7 mm** when injecting **Humulin ® U insulin**; this will make the process easier and prevent needle blockage.

Preparing the insulin

1)   If the **insulin is cloudy**, you should roll the vials between your hands and turn them upside down, to ensure that the contents are mixed thoroughly and that the solution is uniformly cloudy or milky (**do not shake the vial**).

2)   **Disinfect the caps** of the vials containing the cloudy and the clear insulins with an alcohol swab.

3)   **Inject air into the vial of clear insulin.**

> Pull back the plunger of the syringe to draw in a volume of air equal to the amount of clear insulin to be injected. Insert the needle in the rubber cap of the clear insulin vial. Inject the air into the vial. Do not touch the insulin. Withdraw the needle from the vial.

4) Inject the air into the vial of cloudy insulin.

➤ Pull back the plunger on the syringe to draw in enough air to equal your insulin dose. Insert the needle into the rubber cap of the cloudy insulin vial. Inject the air into the vial. Leave the needle in the vial. Do not withdraw the insulin yet.

5) Withdraw the required dose of cloudy insulin.

➤ Turn the cloudy insulin vial and the needle upside down. Pull the plunger back gently in order to draw in the number of units of cloudy insulin required. Withdraw the needle from the vial.

➤ Make sure there are no air bubbles in the syringe; if there are, you may end up injecting a smaller amount of insulin than is required.

➤ Push the plunger until all air bubbles disappear.

➤ Check the syringe to make sure no insulin has been lost; if this is indeed the case, simply replace the missing amount.

6) Prepare the required dose of clear insulin.

➤ Turn the clear insulin vial upside down. Insert the needle into the rubber cap stopper of the clear insulin vial. Do not introduce any cloudy insulin into the clear insulin vial. Pull the plunger back softly in order to draw in the number of clear insulin units to be injected. Withdraw the needle from the vial.

If you have prepared too much clear insulin:

• **discard** the insulin and save the syringe;

• **start** the process over from the very beginning.

In case of contamination of the clear insulin vial by the cloudy insulin:

• **discard** the vial of clear insulin;

• **start** the process over with a new vial.

Injecting of insulin and recording the data

1) **Where to inject the insulin?**

   ➤ Avoid injecting insulin into a limb or part of the body that will be used for an upcoming physical activity (e.g., a leg, if you plan on taking a walk, or an arm, if you intend to play tennis, etc.).

2) **Choose the injection site**, paying special attention to the condition of the skin.

   ➤ Avoid any depression, bump, growth, bruise, blotch or painful spot.

3) **Disinfect the skin** with an alcohol swab or with soap and water and let it dry.

   ➤ Make sure the injection site is clean. At home, it is not absolutely necessary to use alcohol to clean the site – this is optional.

4) **Pinch the skin between your thumb and forefinger and keep pinching it** until the injection is over.

5) Hold the syringe like a pencil and **pierce the skin**.

   ➤ The insulin should be injected into subcutaneous tissue (the tissue beneath the skin).

6) **Inject the insulin** by pushing the plunger all the way down until **all** the insulin has been emptied from the syringe.

   ➤ **Do not pull the plunger back:** If you raise the plunger to check whether or not you hit the right spot, you may damage the skin.

   ➤ **Leave the needle in place** for about **five seconds**.

7) **Withdraw the needle** and delicately press a cotton ball onto the injection site.

8) **Record the number of insulin units** injected as well as the type of insulin used in the appropriate column of your self-monitoring logbook.

5.   What different types of pen injectors are currently available for purchase?

There are several models of pen injectors available on the market (list revised as of July 1, 2004):

Pen injectors	Manufacturers	Cartridges	Graduation	Dosage dial
Huma Pen Ergo®	Eli Lilly Canada Inc.	3 ml	1 unit at a time	1 to 60 units
Pre loaded disposable injectors				
Humulin N Pen®	Eli Lilly Canada Inc.	3 ml	1 unit at a time	1 to 60 units
Humalog Pen®	Eli Lilly Canada Inc.	3 ml	1 unit at a time	1 to 60 units
Humalog Mix 25 Pen®	Eli Lilly Canada Inc.	3 ml	1 unit at a time	1 to 60 units
Novolin-Pen Junior®	Novo Nordisk Canada Inc.	3 ml	0.5 unit at a time	0.5 to 35 units
Novolin-Pen 3®	Novo Nordisk Canada Inc.	3 ml	1 unit at a time	1 to 70 units
Innovo®	Novo Nordisk Canada Inc.	3 ml	1 unit at a time	1 to 70 units
InDuo®	Novo Nordisk Canada Inc. and LifeScan	3 ml	1 unit at a time	1 to 70 units
NovolinSet pre loaded disposable injectors				
Toronto®	Novo Nordisk Canada Inc.	3 ml	2 units at a time	2 to 78 units
30/70®	Novo Nordisk Canada Inc.	3 ml	2 units at a time	2 to 78 units
NPH®	Novo Nordisk Canada Inc.	3 ml	2 units at a time	2 to 78 units

- Check the product monograph for the type of insulin and the type of needle that can be used with the pen injector you choose.

- If you use two types of insulin that have not been premixed, you may use two pen injectors.

6. **How do you prepare and inject insulin when using a pen injector?**

There are three steps in the preparation and injection of insulin with a pen injector.

Preparing the materials

1) **Wash your hands** with soap and water and dry them well.

2) Lay out the **materials**: Pen injector, insulin cartridge, needle, alcohol swab, cotton ball.

    ➤ Use a new needle for each injection.

    ➤ Use an insulin cartridge stored at room temperature.

3) Check the **type and quantity of insulin** remaining in the cartridge.

4) Check the **expiry dates** on the label, namely the date printed by the manufacturer and the date you recorded after opening the cartridge.

    ➤ Do not refrigerate the pen injector: this could damage it or cause air bubbles to form in the cartridge.

    ➤ Do not share a pen injector with another person.

Preparing the insulin

1) **Bring the cloudy insulin to a uniform appearance**. Roll the pen between your palms a dozen times to make sure the cloudy insulin is mixed thoroughly and that it is not stuck to the sides of the cartridge. Next, turn the pen injector over ten times or more. There is a glass marble inside the cartridge containing the cloudy insulin; it will roll from one end of the cartridge to the other, and thus mix the insulin. Do not shake the pen vigorously: this may damage the insulin and reduce its effectiveness.

2) **Fill the empty space in the needle** by injecting one unit of insulin at a time until a drop of insulin appears at the tip of the needle when pointed upwards.

3) **Select the insulin dose to be administered** by turning the dosage dial ring until it reaches the desired number of units.

Injecting insulin and recording the data

1)   Where to inject the insulin.

➤   Avoid injecting insulin into a limb or part of the body that will be used for an upcoming, physical activity (e.g., a leg, if you are going to take a walk or an arm, if you intend to play tennis, etc.).

2)   Choose the injection site, paying special attention to the condition of the skin.

➤   Avoid any depression, bump, growth, bruise, blotch or painful spot.

3)   Disinfect the skin with an alcohol swab or with soap and water and let it dry.

➤   Make sure the injection site is clean. At home, it is not absolutely necessary to use alcohol to clean the site – this is optional.

4)   Pinch the skin between your thumb and forefinger and keep pinching it until the end of the injection if you fit your pen injector with **needles measuring 8 mm to 12 mm**.

5)   It is generally recommended that you do not pinch the skin when using shorter needles (5 mm).

6)   Hold the pen injector like a pencil and **pierce the skin.**

➤   The insulin should be injected into subcutaneous tissue (the tissue beneath the skin).

7)   Push the plunger of the pen injector all the way down so that the **insulin is injected completely.**

➤   **Leave the needle in place** for about **15 seconds.**

8)   Withdraw the needle and delicately press a cotton ball onto the injection site.

➤   **Remove** the needle from the pen injector when the injection is over. Discard the needle.

9)   Record the number of insulin units injected as well as the type of insulin used in the appropriate column of your self-monitoring logbook.

7. What are the recommended techniques for injecting insulin?

As stated earlier, insulin should always be injected into **subcutaneous tissue** (the tissue beneath the skin).

1) Although there is no universal consensus on the best techniques for injecting insulin, there are many proven methods that will help you to self-administer your insulin shots in the safest, gentlest, smoothest and most effective way possible.

2) It is always a good idea to have the process checked by a **healthcare professional** in order to personalize your insulin injection technique. Several factors should be taken into consideration—whether you are a child or an adult, whether you are fat or thin, etc. Another factor to consider is the length of the needle. The need to pinch the skin, and the angle of injection vary from person to person.

> ➤ **For most people, injecting at a 90° angle** allows them to effectively reach subcutaneous tissue. However, **thin people or children** may need to pinch the skin, use short needles or inject at a 45° angle to avoid injecting into muscle tissue, especially in the thigh.

> ➤ **Blood** at the injection site may indicate that you have penetrated a muscle; if so, begin injecting at a 45° angle or use short needles (5 mm and 6 mm).

> ➤ The presence of a **white area** at the site of withdrawal of the needle may indicate that you have not injected the insulin deeply enough.

> ➤ When the technique requires you to squeeze a **fold of skin**, pinch the skin between the thumb and forefinger and be sure to keep pinching it until the injection is finished.

> ➤ When **over 40 units of insulin** have to be injected, better absorption will be achieved by spreading the dose over two injection sites (e.g., the stomach and buttocks).

> ➤ It must be noted that blood glucose levels need to be monitored more closely **if you switch from a long needle to a short one**. Moreover, if you do change needle sizes, you must make sure that insulin absorption remains the same.

CHAPTER 16

Injecting Insulin: Rotation of Injection Sites

1. What are the main areas of the body where insulin may be injected?

Insulin may be injected in different parts of the body. Eight "**injection areas**" are routinely used:

Areas 1 and 2	**ABDOMEN:**	right and left sides, almost everywhere except for 2.5 cm (1 inch) around the navel
Areas 3 and 4	**ARMS:**	anterior-external parts
Areas 5 and 6	**THIGHS:**	anterior-external parts
Areas 7 and 8	**BUTTOCKS:**	fleshy upper parts

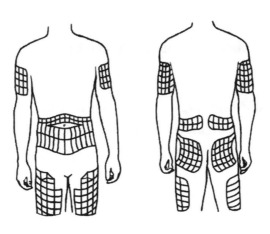

Unless it is possible to locate a fold of skin, it is not advisable to inject the distended abdomen of a pregnant woman, because this can injure the skin.

2.   How many injection sites are there in each area?

In each **injection area**, there are many zones where insulin can be injected; these are called "**injection sites**". You can use the entire surface of each injection area, as long as you observe this principle: do not use **the same injection site more than once a month**.

3.   What distance should be kept between each injection site in the same area?

Each **injection site** in the same area must be at least 1 cm (1/2 inch) away from the site of the previous injection:

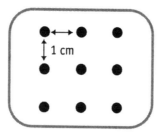

Injection sites

4.   Why must the injection site be changed for each insulin injection?

You must change the injection site **for each insulin injection** to prevent **lipodystrophy** (bumps and cracks from repeated injections at the same site). These subcutaneous deformations may seem unsightly to some, but more important is the fact that they hinder the absorption of insulin and may cause improper control of blood glucose.

5. Is one injection area better than another in terms of insulin absoption?

Yes. For any given type of insulin, the rate of absorption varies according to the injection area used.

The area permitting the fastest absorption is the abdomen, followed by the arms, thighs and buttocks.

Speed of absorption: abdomen > arms > thighs > buttocks

> signifies: greater than

6. What other factors influence the speed of insulin absorption?

Intense exercise increases the rate of insulin absorption provided that you inject the part of your body being exercised.

➡ For example, insulin injected into a thigh is absorbed more quickly if you take a walk or play tennis after the injection.

Other factors such as heat (sun, bath, etc.), the depth of the injection or massaging the injection site can also affect absorption speed.

7. How can I ensure that the amount of insulin absorbed varies as little as possible injection site I use?

To ensure that the amount of insulin absorbed varies as little as possible no matter what injection site you choose, follow these tips and strategies:

1) Inject rapid-acting and short-acting insulin—whether alone or mixed with intermediate-acting insulin—into the **abdomen**. Change the injection site each time you administer your medication.

2) For greater convenience, you can systematically use your upper **arm** to inject rapid-acting or short-acting insulin before lunch. This will ensure that the peak effect of the midday injection will be the same every day, allowing you to adjust the dosage accordingly.

3) Use the **thighs or buttocks** to inject intermediate-acting or long-acting insulin that is not mixed with rapid-acting or short-acting insulin, in order to ensure that absorption is as slow as possible.

4) If multiple injections are administered at different times of the day, it is preferable to use the same injection area of the body at the same time each day.

5) Choose a particular injection area (for speed of absorption) according to a given insulin (time of action) and to the time of injection (activity level).

Example:

Thighs:	slow absorption rate
Humulin® U:	long-acting rate
Bedtime:	reduced activity

To summarize:

Type of insulin	Areas of insulin injection		
	Abdomen	Arm	Thighs and buttocks
Rapid-acting or short-acting, unmixed	Chosen area	Before the midday meal, for convenience	—
Rapid-acting or short-acting and intermediate-acting, mixed	Chosen area	—	—
Intermediate-acting, unmixed	—	—	Chosen area
Long-acting, unmixed	—	—	Chosen area

CHAPTER 17
Storage of Insulin

1. Why must precautions be taken when storing insulin?

Insulin is a fragile product. Insulin solutions and suspensions should be stored according to the manufacturer's recommendations in order to avoid reducing their effectiveness. The use of improperly stored insulin may impair the control of blood glucose.

2. What precautions should be taken when storing insulin?

1) Insulin that is **in use** may be stored for up to one month at room temperature. Injecting cold insulin may cause pain at the injection site.

2) **Supplies of insulin** should be stored in the **refrigerator**. Insulin kept in this manner can be used until the expiry date printed on the label by the manufacturer (commonly referred to as the "best before" date).

3) Insulin must never be directly exposed to sunlight or heat. You may not be able to tell the insulin has been altered just by looking at it, since these conditions do not necessarily change the appearance of the product. Insulin exposed to excessive heat must be discarded.

4) Insulin must never be frozen. Freezing does not always change the appearance of the product. Insulin that has been frozen must be discarded.

5) A pen injector must not be stored in the refrigerator; this could damage it or create air bubbles in the cartridge.

6)   Spare insulin syringes prepared in advance should be kept in the refrigerator, stored in an uprigh or slightly slanted position, with the needle (and its cap) always pointing upwards. This will prevent insulin particles from clogging the needle.

7)   It is important to record the date the insulin was opened in the space provided on the container.

8)   Always store reserve insulin in the refrigerator, e.g., in case of breakage.

3.   What are some specific recommendations for the storage of insulin?

The following table shows the temperatures and storage times recommended by insulin manufacturers, according to the formats and brands they make available.

Format	Brand	Recommended temperature	Maximum duration of storage
Unopened vial or cartridge	Humulin ® Humalog ®	2°C-8°C	Expiry date on the container
	Novolin ® NovoRapid ®	2°C-10°C	Expiry date on the container
Opened vial	Humulin ®	18°C-25°C (max. 25°C)	1 month
	Humalog ®	18°C-25°C (max. 30°C)	1 month
	Novolin ®	18°C-25°C (max. 25°C)	1 month
	NovoRapid ®	18°C-25°C (max. 37°C)	1 month

Format	Brand	Recommended temperature	Maximum duration of storage
Opened cartridge	Humulin®	18°C-25°C (max. 25°C)	1 month
	Humalog®	18°C-25°C (max. 30°C)	1 month
	Novolin® NovoRapid®	18°C-25°C (max. 37°C)	1 month
Preloaded disposable pen injector unopened	Humulin® N Pen Humalog® Pen	2°C-8°C	Expiry date on the container
	NovolinSet®	2°C-10°C	Expiry date on the container
Preloaded disposable pen injector opened	Humulin® N Pen	18°C-25°C (max. 25°C)	1 month
	Humalog® Pen	18°C-25°C (max. 30°C)	1 month
	NovolinSet®	18°C-25°C (max. 37°C)	1 month
Syringe prepared in advance	Humulin® Humalog®	2°C-8°C	3 weeks
	Novolin® NovoRapid®	2°C-10°C	Use as quickly as possible

4. What should insulin look like?

Insulin may come in a **clear** solution that resembles water, or in an opaque suspension that is **cloudy** or milky.

Clear insulins		Cloudy insulins	
Rapid-acting:	Humalog ® NovoRapid ®	*Intermediate-acting:*	Humulin ® N Novolin ® ge NPH Humulin ® L
Short-acting:	Humulin ® R Novolin ® ge Toronto	*Long-acting:*	Humulin ® U
Long-acting:	Lantus ®	*Premixed:*	Humulin ® 30/70 Humalog ® Mix 25 Novolin ® ge 10/90 Novolin ® ge 20/80 Novolin ® ge 30/70 Novolin ® ge 40/60 Novolin ® ge 50/50

5.   When should clear insulin be discarded?

Clear insulin must be discarded if:

➤   it looks cloudy or milky;

➤   it is thick;

➤   it contains solid particles;

➤   it has been exposed to extreme temperatures (heat or cold);

➤   the recommended "best before date" has expired.

6.   What precautions should be taken with cloudy insulin?

Cloudy insulin is a suspension that must be **mixed well** before being used.

The presence of a whitish deposit at the bottom of the vial or in the cartridge is normal, but it must be remixed into the suspension by rolling the vial between your palms and turning it upside down, or by turning the cartridge over in the pen injector several times. **Do not shake them.**

Insulin should have a uniform appearance.

You have to be particularly meticulous when you are preparing a mix of long-acting insulin (Humulin® U).

An inadequate mix of cloudy insulin may alter the precision of measured insulin doses.

7. When should cloudy insulin be discarded?

Cloudy insulin should be discarded if:

- ➤ a deposit remains at the bottom of the vial or in cartridge;
- ➤ there are specks floating in the insulin;
- ➤ particles are stuck to the side of the vial or cartridge, making these containers look frosty;
- ➤ it has been exposed to extreme temperatures (of heat or cold);
- ➤ the recommended "best before" date has expired.

CHAPTER 18

Adjustment of Insulin Doses

1. Why should insulin doses be adjusted?

Insulin treatments are adjusted to improve the control of blood glucose levels. Ideally, people with diabetes should learn how to adjust insulin doses on their own, after having received the appropriate information from a healthcare team.

2. Which blood glucose levels should be the targets when adjusting insulin doses?

The majority of people with diabetes should aim for blood glucose levels between 4 mmol/l and 7 mmol/l before meals, and between 5 mmol/l and 10 mmol/l one or two hours after meals. However, if there is no risk, you can aim for normal blood glucose levels, that is, between 4 mmol/l and 6 mmol/l before meals and between 5 mmol/l and 8 mmol/l one or two hours after meals.

3. What are the rules for adjusting insulin doses?

The following rules are a guide to help you make decisions regarding your insulin dose adjustments. They will help to ensure that the adjustments you make will be safe and effective.

These are the basic principles you should be aware of:

➤   insulin lowers blood glucose levels and;

➤   the current blood glucose level reflects what happened before.

Before adjusting insulin doses, it is important to take the time to analyze blood glucose levels by calculating the average of your last three readings for each period of the day (morning, noon, evening and bedtime) without going back more than seven days. Only take into consideration readings taken since the previous adjustment.

Here are the six rules for adjusting insulin doses:

1)   In your calculations, do not include any measurement below 4 mmol/l or above 7 mmol/l associated with a **situation that is sporadic, exceptional or attributable to an isolated cause.**

2)   Never adjust your insulin dose on the basis of **one blood glucose test only.** It is generally not recommended that you adjust a dose to correct an immediate blood glucose level.

3)   Always adjust **only one insulin dose** at a time.

4)   First correct the **hypoglycemic situations**, starting with the first one of the day, then the second, etc.

➤   We are dealing with a **hypoglycemic situation** if:

•   the average level is below 4 mmol/l during the same period of any given day;

•   during the same period of any given day you observe two hypoglycemic readings among the last two taken, or you note three non-consecutive hypoglycemic readings over the last seven days, even if their average is greater than or equal to 4 mmol/l.

➤   Assign a value of 2 mmol/l to any hypoglycemia that has not been measured.

➤ A hypoglycemic reading taken outside the four usual blood glucose measuring times should be recorded for the following period (e.g., record your morning hypoglycemic reading in the "before lunch" column).

5) Afterwards, correct **hyperglycemic situations**, that is, these producing reading that, on average, are greater than 7 mmol/l for the same period of the day.

➤ Watch out for **rebound hyperglycemia**, which is a situation following hypoglycemic episodes during which blood glucose levels rise **above 7 mmol/l**. Hyperglycemic episodes need not be taken into consideration when calculating average levels. Nocturnal hypoglycemia may cause rebound hyperglycemia upon waking. When in doubt, take a blood glucose reading around 2 a.m. and if hypoglycemia is observed, correct this condition rather than the morning hyperglycemia.

6) Wait at least two days after an insulin adjustment before introducing any more modifications. Wait at least three days if the adjustment concerns a long-acting insulin. The only exception to this rule would occur in the event of two consecutive hypoglycemic readings. In that case, disregard the rule and decrease the dose of the responsible insulin.

4. What are the most frequently used insulin regimens?

There are several insulin regimens; here are four of the most commonly prescribed ones.

1) The **"split-mixed" regimen** consists of taking an insulin injection before breakfast and before dinner. Each injection consists of a combination of intermediate-acting (e.g., Humulin® N or Novolin® ge NPH) insulin and either rapid-acting (Humalog® or NovoRapid®) or short-acting (Humulin® R or Novolin® ge Toronto) insulin. Sometimes, the injection of the intermediate-acting insulin before dinner must be delayed until bedtime to prevent nocturnal hypoglycemia.

2)   The **"multiple daily injections (MDI)" regimen** consists of injecting one rapid-acting (Humalog® or NovoRapid®) or short-acting (Humulin® R or Novolin® ge Toronto) insulin before each meal and one intermediate-acting (e.g., Humulin® N or Novolin® ge NPH) or long-acting (Humulin® U) insulin at bedtime. Although basal insulin is usually administered in one injection, it can also be taken in several injections throughout the course of the day. The rapid-acting or short-acting insulin dose may be fixed (fixed carbohydrate regimen) or set according to the amount of carbohydrates consumed during a meal (variable carbohydrate regimen). In the variable carbohydrate regimen, the dose is determined in terms of a ratio, for example 1 unit/10 g of carbohydrates, that is, 1 unit of insulin per 10 g of carbohydrates consumed.

3)   The **"premixed" regimen** consists of injecting a premixed insulin (e.g., Humulin® 30/70, Novolin® ge 30/70, Novolin® ge 50/50, Humalog® Mix 25, etc.) before breakfast and dinner.

4)   The **"combined" regimen** consists of injecting one intermediate-acting (Humulin® N or Novolin® ge NPH) insulin or long-acting (Humulin® U) insulin at bedtime, along with the usual oral antidiabetic medications taken during the day.

5.   In the " split-mixed " regimen, which insulins affect blood glucose levels during of the day?

Insulin in use:	affects	blood glucose levels:
intermediate-acting before dinner	———▶	before breakfast
rapid- or short-acting before breakfast	———▶	before lunch
intermediate-acting before breakfast	———▶	before dinner
rapid- or short-acting before dinner	———▶	at bedtime

Remember: your blood glucose level reading at any given time will reflect the effects of your last insulin injection.

6.   How should insulin doses be adjusted in the "split-mixed" regimen?

In general, when faced with a **hypoglycemic situation (blood glucose average below 4 mmol/l)** before meals and at bedtime (as defined in the adjustment rules), you must **decrease** the dose of the responsible insulin by two units at a time. However, if the **total daily dose** of insulin is less than or equal to 20 units, reduce the dose by one unit at a time.

Generally, when facing a **hyperglycemic situation (blood glucose average above 7 mmol/l)** before meals and at bedtime (as defined in the adjustment rules), you must **increase** the dose of the responsible insulin by two units at a time. However, if the **total daily dose** of insulin is less than or equal to 20 units, increase the dose by one unit at a time.

It is advisable to wait at least two days before making any changes in your insulin doses. In case of hypoglycemic or hyperglycemic situations, do not wait any longer than a week to adjust the dose of the responsible insulin.

7.   In the "multiple daily injections (MDI)" regimen, which insulins affect blood glucose levels during the day?

Insulin in use:	affects	blood glucose levels:
intermediate- or long-acting at bedtime	⟶	before breakfast
rapid- or short-acting before breakfast	⟶	before lunch
rapid- or short-acting before lunch	⟶	before dinner
rapid- or short-acting before dinner	⟶	at bedtime

Remember: your blood glucose level reading at any given time will reflect the effects of your last insulin injection.

8. How should insulin doses be adjusted in the "multiple daily injections (MDI)" regimen in conjunction with a fixed carbohydrate plan?

In general, when faced with a **hypoglycemic situation (blood glucose average below 4 mmol/l)** before meals and at bedtime (as defined in the adjustment rules), you must **decrease** the dose of the responsible insulin by two units at a time. However, if the **total daily dose** of insulin is less than or equal to 20 units, reduce the dose by one unit at a time.

Generally, when faced with a **hyperglycemic situation (blood glucose average above 7 mmol/l)** before meals and at bedtime (as defined in the adjustment rules), you must **increase** the dose of the responsible insulin by two units at a time. However, if the **total daily dose** of insulin is less than or equal to 20 units, increase the dose by one unit at a time.

It is advisable to wait at least two days before making any adjustments to the doses of rapid-acting (Humalog® or NovoRapid®), short-acting (Humulin® R or Novolin® ge Toronto) or intermediate-acting (e.g., Humulin® N or Novolin® ge NPH) insulin. However, if a dose of long-acting insulin (Humulin® U) has been adjusted, you must wait at least three days before adjusting any new dose of insulin (long-, rapid-or short-acting). The only exception to this rule is if two consecutive hypoglycemic episodes occur in the same period; in this case, ignore the rule and decrease the dose of the responsible insulin. In the case of hypoglycemic or hyperglycemic situations, never wait more than a week to adjust the insulin.

9. How should insulin doses be adjusted in the "multiple daily injections (MDI)" regimen in conjunction with a variable carbohydrate?

When faced with a **hypoglycemic situation (blood glucose average below 4 mmol/l)**, as defined in the previous rules of adjustment:

1) during the night or before breakfast, you must **decrease** the dose of intermediate-acting (e.g., Humulin® N or Novolin® ge NPH) or long-acting

(Humulin® U) insulin by two units at a time. However, if the daily dose of intermediate-acting or long-acting insulin is less than or equal to 10 units, decrease the dose one unit at a time;

2) before lunch, dinner or bedtime, you must **decrease** the dose of the responsible insulin (Humalog®, NovoRapid®, Humulin® R or Novolin® ge Toronto) by 0.2 units/10 g of carbohydrates. However, if the dose of this insulin is less than or equal to 0.5 units/10 g of carbohydrates, decrease the dose by only 0.1 unit/10 g of carbohydrates at a time.

In a **hyperglycemic situation (blood glucose average above 7 mmol/l)**, as defined in the rules of adjustment:

1) during the night or before breakfast, you must **increase** the dose of intermediate-acting (e.g., Humulin® N or Novolin® ge NPH) or long-acting (Humulin® U) insulin by two units at a time. However, if the daily dose of intermediate-acting or long-acting insulin is less than or equal to 10 units, increase the dose one unit at a time;

2) before lunch, dinner or bedtime, you must **increase** the dose of the responsible insulin (Humalog®, NovoRapid®, Humulin® R or Novolin® ge Toronto) by 0.2 units/10 g of carbohydrates. However, if the dose of this insulin is less than or equal to 0.5 units/10 g of carbohydrates, increase the dose by only 0.1 unit/10 g of carbohydrates at a time.

It is recommended that you wait at least two days before making any adjustments of doses of rapid-acting (Humalog® or NovoRapid®), short-acting (Humulin® R or Novolin® ge Toronto) or intermediate-acting (e.g., Humulin® N or Novolin® ge NPH) insulin. However, if a dose of long-acting insulin (Humulin® U) has already been adjusted, you must wait at least three days before adjusting any new dose of insulin (long-, rapid- or short-acting). The only exception to this rule is if two consecutive bouts of hypoglycemia occur in the same period; in this case, ignore the rule and decrease the dose of the responsible insulin. In the case of hypoglycemic or hyperglycemic situations, never wait more than a week to adjust the insulin.

10. In the "premixed" regimen, which insulins affect blood glucose levels during of the day?

Premixed insulin:	affects	blood glucose levels:
rapid- or short-acting and intermediate-acting before breakfast	———▶	before lunch and dinner
rapid- or short-acting and intermediate-acting before dinner	———▶	at bedtime and before breakfast

Remember: your blood glucose level reading at any given time will reflect the effects of your last insulin injection.

11. How should insulin doses be adjusted in the "premixed" regimen?

In general, when faced with a **hypoglycemic situation (blood glucose average below 4 mmol/l)** before meals and at bedtime (as defined in the adjustment rules), you must **decrease** the dose of the responsible mixed insulin by two units at a time. However, if the **total daily dose** of insulin is less than or equal to 20 units, reduce the dose by one unit at a time.

In general, when facing a **hyperglycemic situation (blood glucose average above 7 mmol/l),** as defined by the adjustment rules, you must **increase** the mixed dose of the responsible insulin by two units at a time. However, if the **total daily dose** of insulin is less than or equal to 20 units, increase the dose by one unit at a time.

Remember that premixed insulins cover two daily periods at a time. As a result, if there is a marked difference between blood glucose levels at bedtime and in the morning (e.g., they are high at bedtime and low in the morning) or between those before lunch and before dinner, you must **see your doctor, because this contrast may indicate that the insulin mixture must be changed.**

It is advisable to wait at least two days before making any new adjustment of your insulin doses. In case of hypoglycemic or hyperglycemic situations, never wait more than one week to adjust the dose of the responsible insulin.

12. In the "combined" regimen, which blood glucose reading is affected by insulin administered at bedtime?

In the "combined" regimen, **morning blood glucose** is affected by intermediate-acting or long-acting insulin administered at bedtime.

13. How should insulin doses be adjusted in the "combined" regimen?

In general, when faced with **hypoglycemic situation in the morning (blood glucose average below 4 mmol/l)**, as defined in the adjustment rules, you must **decrease** the bedtime insulin dose by two units at a time. However, if the total daily dose of insulin is less than or equal to 10 units, reduce the dose by one unit.

In general, when facing a morning **hyperglycemic situation (blood glucose average above 7 mmol/l)**, as defined by the adjustment rules, you must **increase** the bedtime insulin dose by two units at a time. However, if the total daily dose of insulin is less than or equal to 10 units, increase the dose by one unit.

It is advisable to wait at least two days before making any new adjustments to the intermediate-acting insulin and three days for the long-acting insulin. In case of hypoglycemic or hyperglycemic situations, never wait more than one week to adjust the dose of the responsible insulin.

A few practical examples of adjustments

Before you adjust insulin doses yourself, it is important that you understand the adjustment rules that we have described in this chapter. Here are several examples of their application:

Example no. 1

Treatment: "Split-mixed" regimen

Humulin® R	12 units at breakfast and 10 units at dinner
Humulin® N	20 units at breakfast and 14 units at dinner
Total daily dose of insulin = 56 units	

Self-monitoring logbook

Date	BLOOD GLUCOSE			
	Before breakfast (mmol/l)	Before lunch (mmol/l)	Before dinner (mmol/l)	At bedtime (mmol/l)
16/05	6.4	7.7	6.5	5.7
17/05	7.1	9.3	7.0	5.4
18/05	5.9	7.5	6.2	6.0
Average	6.5	8.2	6.6	5.7

Analysis

We can see that the average blood glucose level before lunch is greater than 7 mmol/l (hyperglycemia). The appropriate adjustment in this situation would be to **increase** short-acting insulin in the morning by two units.

Example no. 2

Treatment: "Multiple daily injections (MDI)" regimen with a fixed carbohydrate plan

NovoRapid®	8 units at breakfast, 6 units at lunch, 6 units at dinner
Novolin® ge NPH	16 units at bedtime
Total daily dose of insulin = 36 units	

Self-monitoring logbook

Date	BLOOD GLUCOSE			
	Before breakfast (mmol/l)	Before lunch (mmol/l)	Before dinner (mmol/l)	At bedtime (mmol/l)
03/01	12.0	9.0	8.0	6.5
04/01	13.0	8.7	7.2	5.8
05/01	11.7	8.9	7.8	5.6
Average	12.2	8.9	7.7	6.0

Analysis

Here we notice a hyperglycemic situation occurring before breakfast, lunch and dinner. To start, we will correct the first hyperglycemic period of the day, before breakfast. To do so, we should **increase** the dose of NPH insulin taken at bedtime to 18 units. Before making this adjustment, it would be a good idea to **check blood glucose** at 2 a.m. in order to eliminate nocturnal hypoglycemia, which could cause an episode of rebound hyperglycemia in the morning. If in fact there is hypoglycemia at night, the bedtime NPH insulin should instead be **decreased** by 2 units.

Example no 3

Treatment: "multiple daily injections (MDI)" regimen with a variable carbohydrate plan

Humalog ®	1.2 units/10 g of carbohydrates at breakfast
	1.0 unit/10 g of carbohydrates at lunch
	0.8 units/10 g of carbohydrates at dinner
Humulin ® U	12 units at bedtime

Self-monitoring logbook

Date	BLOOD GLUCOSE			
	Before breakfast (mmol/l)	Before lunch (mmol/l)	Before dinner (mmol/l)	At bedtime (mmol/l)
13/04	5.4	6.4	4.4	5.8
14/04	5.9	6.0	3.6	5.0
15/04	5.3	5.6	2.8	5.2
Average	5.5	6.0	3.6	5.3

Analysis

We can see by looking at the chart above that two **hypoglycemic episodes** were revealed by the last two blood glucose readings taken before dinner. The appropriate adjustment, then would be to **decrease** insulin before lunch by 0.2 units/10 g of carbohydrates, thus from 1.0 unit/10 g to 0.8 units/10 g of carbohydrates.

CHAPTER 19

The Insulin Pump:

Another Option for the Treatment of Diabetes

1. What is an insulin pump?

An insulin pump is a device consisting of:

1) a reservoir or cartridge containing insulin;

2) an electric motor to inject insulin from the reservoir;

3) a catheter (cannula) attached to the insulin reservoir that is equipped with a small needle for injecting insulin beneath the skin of the abdomen.

An insulin pump allows insulin to be administered subcutaneously on a continuous basis, 24 hours a day; this is called the **basal rate**. The basal rate supplies all insulin needs regardless of mealtimes (basal dose). The pump may be programmed to provide different basal rates in order to respond to varied insulin needs during different periods of the day. Before meals, the pump can be used to deliver a supplemental dose to meet the insulin needs associated with meals; this is called the **bolus dose**. Together, the continual release of insulin and the pre-meal bolus imitate the normal function of the pancreas.

Nowadays, it is recommended to use a rapid-acting insulin such as Humalog® or NovoRapid® with the insulin pump.

The insulin pump is not an artificial pancreas. It does only what it is programmed to do.

2.   What are some basic guidelines for using an insulin pump?

Current guidelines on the use of insulin pumps have a tendency to be somewhat restrictive because of the treatments cost. Here are some commonly recognized guidelines and indications for the use of insulin pumps:

1)   for serious hypoglycemia (requiring the help of another person) on more than one occasion (two or more episodes over the course of the last 12 months);

2)   for marked variations in blood glucose readings, requiring repeated medical attention (two or more hospitalizations over the last 12 months);

3)   for inadequate control of blood glucose (glycosylated hemoglobin greater than or equal to 7%) despite attempts to control it with intensive insulinotherapy;

4)   in case of rapid progression of complications (such as retinopathy and/or neuropathy) with only sub-optimal control of blood glucose levels (glycosylated hemoglobin greater than 8%).

The insulin pump may also be an option in the following cases:

1)   pregnancy;

2)   when someone is willing to use a pump and is capable of covering the costs of the treatment.

3.   What are the costs of an insulin-pump treatment?

An insulin pump costs about $6,000 and the materials required (needles, catheters, insulin, etc.) can cost between $2,000 and $4,000 a year.

4.   Does the Régime d'assurance médicaments of the gouvernement of Québec cover the costs of an insulin pump?

No. The Régime d'assurance médicaments of Québec does not cover the cost related to the purchase of an insulin pump or of the required materials. However, some private insurance companies cover up to 80% of the costs if treatment is justified.

5.   How can I find out if an insulin pump is for me?

First, discuss the matter with your endocrinologist. If insulin pump treatment is appropriate for you, you must:

1)   ask your insurance company if it covers the treatment costs related to an insulin pump;

2)   get from your doctor:

   ➤   a prescription for an insulin pump;

   ➤   a letter justifying insulin pump treatment, which will be sent to your insurance company.

6.   What procedures should be followed when using an insulin pump?

Using an insulin pump requires some instruction which should be provided by a qualified healthcare team.

Your endocrinologist will prescribe insulin doses and ajust them, if necessary. You must learn:

1)   how the pump functions;

2)   how to install the catheter and how to choose the injection area;

3)   how to calculate carbohydrates;

4)   how to adjust your insulin doses by yourself.

Ask your endocrinologist about procedures you should follow and the people you should contact.

7.   How is insulin dose required for an insulin pump determined?

As a rule, rapid-acting insulin (Humalog® or NovoRapid®) is used for insulin pumps.

To determine the correct **basal dose**, it is recommended to begin with 50% of the total dose of insulin required for the day, based on the most recent daily treatment (for example: total dose for 24 hours = 40 units, so 40 ÷ 2 = 20 units for the basal dose). When determining the daily distribution of the basal dose: two important facts should be taken into consederation, in general, the 12 a.m. to 4 a.m. period is the period most sensitive to insulin and therefore the time when a person is most vulnerable to hypoglycemia. By contrast, the 4 a.m. to 8 a.m. period is the most resistant to insulin, and thus generally requires more insulin. Therefore, it is a good idea to decrease the midnight basal rate by 25% and increase the 4 a.m. rate by 50%.

For instance, if the insulin dose were 20 units per 24 hours, the basal rate would be 0.8 units per hour (20 units ÷ 24 hours = 0.8 units per hour). However, because of the factors mentioned above the basal rate between midnight and 4 a.m. would most likely be reduced by 25% (to 0.6 units per hour) and the rate between 4 a.m. and 8 a.m., increased by 50% (to 1.2 units per hour).

To determine the **pre-meal bolus insulin dose,** one could begin with 1.0 unit per 10 g of carbohydrates for each meal, then adjust the dose according to the person's needs. For example, a meal containing 60 g of carbohydrates requires a dose of 6 units: (60 g ÷ 10 g) x 1,0 unit = 6 units.

8.   Do several basal rates have to be programmed during the day?

Not necessarily. However, since a day comprises five distinct periods that may require different basal rates, these should be adjusted accordingly.

Period 1: 12 a.m.–4 a.m. Period during which hypoglycemia is most likely to occur and in which less insulin or a lower basal rate may be used.

Period 2: 4 a.m.–8 a.m. Period when insulin resistance can create a need for more insulin or for a higher basal rate.

Period 3: 8 a.m.–12 p.m. Active period during the day that can require a lower basal rate.

Period 4: 12 a.m.–6 p.m. Active period during the day that can require a lower basal rate.

Period 5: 6 p.m.–12 a.m. Less active period that can require a higher basal rate.

9.   Which blood glucose readings indicate that basal rate adjustments should be made?

It is important to identify your blood glucose readings during the day and their corresponding basal rates from each time period, to see whether these require any adjustments.

Period		Basal blood glucose
12 a.m. to 4 a.m.	⟶	2 a.m.
4 to 8 a.m.	⟶	before breakfast (about 7–8 a.m.)
8 a.m. to 12 p.m.	⟶	before lunch (about 11 a.m.–12 p.m.)
12 p.m. to 6 p.m.	⟶	before dinner (about 4–6 p.m.)
6 p.m. to 12 a.m.	⟶	bedtime (about 11 p.m.–12 a.m.)

10. Which blood glucose readings indicate that adjustments to pre-meal bolus doses should be made?

The bolus for each meal should be adjusted according to the blood glucose reading taken after the meal (one or two hours after).

Meal		Postprandial blood glucose (1 or 2 hours after a meal)
Breakfast	⟶	after breakfast
Lunch	⟶	after lunch
Dinner	⟶	after dinner

11. What are blood glucose targets?

Basal blood glucose:

For most people, it is recommended to aim for blood glucose levels that are between 4 mmol/l and 7 mmol/l before meals and at bedtime (before the snack). However, if there is no risk, it is suggested to aim for normal blood glucose levels, that is, those between 4 mmol/l and 6 mmol/l before meals and at bedtime (before the snack).

Postprandial blood glucose:

It is advisable to aim for a blood glucose level after a meal that is higher than the level before it. Furthermore, most people should aim for a postprandial blood glucose level that is between 5 mmol/l and 10 mmol/l (one or two hours after a meal). However, if there is no risk, it is suggested to aim for normal blood glucose, that is, between 5 mmol/l and 8 mmol/l one or two hours after a meal.

12. What are the rules for adjusting insulin doses?

Before adjusting insulin doses, it is important to take the time to analyze blood glucose levels by calculating the average of the last two or three readings for each period of the day (before meals, after meals and at bedtime), without going back any further than seven days. Only use readings taken since the last adjustment.

Here are the six rules for adjusting insulin doses:

1) In your calculations, do not include any measurement below 4 mmol/l or above 7 mmol/l associated with a **situation that is sporadic, exceptional or attributable to an isolated cause.**

2) Never adjust your insulin dose on the basis of **one blood glucose test only.** It is generally not recommended to adjust your dose to correct an immediate blood glucose level.

3) Always adjust **only one insulin** dose at a time (basal rate or bolus), during only one period of the day.

4) First correct **hypoglycemic situations,** starting with the first one of the day.

   ➤ We are dealing with a **basal hypoglycemic situation** if:
   - the basal blood glucose average is below 4 mmol/l during the same period of the day;
   - during the same period of the day, there are two hypoglycemic readings among the two last glucose readings taken, or if three non-consecutive hypoglycemic readings have been noticed over the last seven days, even if their average is greater than or equal to 4 mmol/l.

   ➤ We are dealing with a **postprandial hypoglycemic situation** if:
   - the average postprandial blood glucose reading taken after a meal is lower than the average blood glucose reading taken before the same meal;
   - for the same meal time, there are two postprandial hypoglycemic readings among the last two taken, or if three non-consecutive hypoglycemic readings have been taken over the last seven days, which are below the blood glucose level noted before the meal. This applies even if the average postprandial blood glucose level is higher than the average blood glucose level before the meal.

   ➤ Assign a value of 2 mmol/l to any hypoglycemic episode that has not been measured.

➤ A hypoglycemic reading taken outside the four usual blood glucose measuring periods should be recorded as data for the closest following time period closest to it, in your logbook (e.g., a hypoglycemic reading measured at 11 a.m. should be written down in the "before lunch" column).

5) Afterwards, correct the **hyperglycemic situations**. That is to say, those readings which indicate a basal blood glucose average of over 7 mmol/l for a given period of the day, or an average that is over 10 mmol/l for postprandial blood glucose. As always, perform your corrections in sequence, beginning with the first day, then the second, etc.

- Watch out for **rebound hyperglycemia**. A basal blood glucose level that is higher that 7 mmol/l, and which follows a hypoglycemic episode, is known as rebound hyperglycemia. This hyperglycemic reading need not be taken into account when calculating the average.

6) Wait at least two days after an adjustment before making any other modifications.

13. How should insulin doses be adjusted?

On the basis of blood glucose readings taken at 2 a.m., before meals and at bedtime for the basal rate; and, finally, for blood glucose measured one or two hours after meals for the bolus doses, you should adjust your insulin doses as follows:

➤ Basal rate:

- In case of *hypoglycemia* ➔ **decrease** the corresponding basal rate by 0.1 units/hour to 0.2 units/hour.
- In case of *hyperglycemia* ➔ **increase** the corresponding basal rate by 0.1 units/hour to 0.2 units/hour.

➤ Bolus:

- In case of *hypoglycemia* ➔ **decrease** the bolus by 0.1 units/10 g of carbohydrates to 0.2 units/10 g of carbohydrates.
- In case of *hyperglycemia* ➔ **increase** the bolus by 0.1 units/10 g to 0.2 units/10 g of carbohydrates.

14. Which insulin pumps are available in Canada?

Here is a list of the latest commercially available insulin pumps, with a few of their characteristics (list revised as of July 1, 2004, adapted from www.insulinpumps.cc)

The choice of an insulin pump should be discussed with your doctor and with an insulin pump specialist.

Manufacturer	Auto Control Medical	Smiths Medical Canada	Medtronic MiniMed
Name	Animas ® IR 1000	Deltec Cozmo ®	Paradigm 512 ®
Appearance Dimensions in cm	9.0 x 5.5 x 2.0	8.0 x 4.7 x 2.4	5 x 7.6 x 2.0
Size in cubic cm	99.0	90.0	76.0
Available colours	dark grey, or various colours	ice blue, dark grey	clear, blue, charcoal, violet
Weight of pump	116 g	90 g	90 g
Operational components Cartridge insulin capacity	300 units	300 units	176 units (300 U/model 712)
Catheters interchangeable with other pumps	yes	yes	no
Screen backlight	yes	yes	yes
Waterproofness	yes	yes	water resistant
Bolus characteristics Dosage per cycles	0.1 units	0.05 units or program 0.10, 0.20, 0.50 and 1.0 units	0.1 units

Manufacturer	Auto Control Medical	Smiths Medical Canada	Medtronic MiniMed
Name	Animas ® IR 1000	Deltec Cozmo ®	Paradigm 512 ®
Bolus calculator	no	no	yes
Audible alert	yes; two volume levels	yes; two volume levels plus vibration option	yes; 2 to 4 units
Bolus duration per unit	3 seconds	1 to 5 minutes	40 seconds
Long bolusyes	yes	yes	
Combined bolus (duo)	no	yes	yes
Audible reminder of blood glucose reading after bolus	no	yes	yes
Remote control	no	no	yes (optional)
Memory	last 255 days	2,000 events and/ or, 90 last days	last 24 boluses on screen (90 days on software)
Basal rate characteristics			
Rate per profile	12	48	48
Number of profile	4	4	3
Temporary basal rate	yes; by percentage	yes; by percentage or by units of insulin	yes; by percentage or by fixed value
Programmed dosage	0.05 units/h.	0.05 units/h.	0.05 units/h.
Dosage delivery	doses injected every 3 min.	doses injected every 3 min.	Hourly rate delivered by precise pulses of 0.05 units distributed evenly over the hour
Other components			
Downloadable	coming soon	yes	yes (with optional software)

Manufacturer	Auto Control Medical	Smiths Medical Canada	Medtronic MiniMed
Name	Animas ® IR 1000	Deltec Cozmo ®	Paradigm 512 ®
Emergency pump availabilitypump the	replacement pump the next day	replacement pump the next day	replacement next day
Meter which sends glucose readings to pump	no	no	yes Paradigm Link ®
Cost of pump*	$6,400	$6,000 (includes software and infrared adaptor)	$6,400 (includes pump and Paradigm Link® glucose meter which sends glucose readings to pump by radio waves, RF)
Update of pump	no	no	yes, optional, for duration of 4-year guarantee; "Paradigm Pathway" program
Batteries	Four 1.5 V, model 357; last 6 to 8 weeks; ≃ $8/month	one AAA alkaline; lasts about 30 days in audible mode, less in vibration mode; ≃ $4 to $8/month	one AAA alkaline; lasts 1-3 weeks; ≃ $4/month
Ease of programming– menus like "Windows"	yes	yes	yes

* Prices subject to change. Accompanying supplies for an insulin pump can cost between $2,000 and $4,000 a year.

Manufacturer	Auto Control Medical	Smiths Medical Canada	Medtronic MiniMed
Name	Animas ® IR 1000	Deltec Cozmo ®	Paradigm 512 ®
Memory	bolus recall, alarm, and daily insulin total for last 255 days, including date and time	recall of 4,000 data for last 90 days	recall of 24 last boluses (detailed history: blood glucose, carbohydrates, type of bolus, dosage, date, hour, etc.); recall of 36 alarms, 20 purges and daily total from last 14 days (90 days on software)
Help line	1 800 463-5414	1 800 826-9703	1 800 217-1617
Website	www.animascorp.com	www.delteccozmo.com	www.minimed.com

CHAPTER 20
Physical Activity

1. What is physical activity?

All bodily movement produced by the muscles and requiring an increase in energy expenditure, may be defined as physical activity.

2. Why is it important to get regular exercise?

Whether we have **diabetes or not**, regular exercise is essential and beneficial to our health. All regular exercise:

1) improves physical fitness, posture, balance, self-esteem and stress management;

2) helps control weight and decrease fat levels in blood;

3) helps prevent diseases such as high blood pressure, diabetes, heart disease, circulatory problems and osteoporosis;

4) increases life expectancy.

3. What are the benefits of a regular exercise program for people who are glucose intolerant (pre-diabetic) or for those with diabetes?

People with glucose intolerance and those with diabetes derive the same benefits from exercise as people with normal glucose tolerance. Furthermore, for people with glucose intolerance, moderate regular physical activity decreases the risk of developing diabetes. For people with type 2 diabetes, regular physical activity decreases resistance to insulin and thus helps to better control diabetes.

Regular exercise is as beneficial to a person with type 1 diabetes as it is to someone who does not have the disease. However, it is vital that the person with diabetes control his or her illness and adjust insulin doses and diet according to the physical activity involved.

4.   How can I find an exercise program that I can stick to?

1)   First of all, choose a sport or activity you like. Dancing, light gymnastics, swimming, working out at the gym, walking at a fast pace, etc., are all examples of simple and practical physical activities. The important thing is to decide on a sport or activity that you truly enjoy. This will increase the likelihood that you will exercise on a daily basis.

2)   Include the activity in your daily schedule. The more regularly a person exercises, the better he or she will feel. Our daily schedules usually offer any number of opportunities for exercise, which might include:

➤   walking or biking to work;

➤   taking the stairs rather than the elevator;

➤   doing some work around the house or yard such as sweeping, cleaning windows, gardening, etc.

In order to reap real health benefits, your exercise program should allow you to burn 1,000 to 1,500 extra calories per week. There are a number of ways to reach this goal, depending on the type of activity involved, as well as its intensity, duration and frequency.

The following table (taken from a 1999 release of the Scientific Committee of Kino-Québec) offers guidelines concerning the frequency and duration of the physical activity (sorted by level of intensity) required to burn 1,000 calories per week.

Intensity (level)	Frequency (number of times per week)	Duration (minutes)	Calories per session
Low	7	60	150
	4	90 to 120	250
Moderate	7	30	150
	4	45	250
Elevated	7	20	150
	4	30	250

5. What are the hallmarks of a physical fitness program that can help control diabetes?

A good exercise program includes the following:

1) The exercises require **moderate effort levels**.

2) The exercises can be done most days of the week — **at least five days a week**.

3) The person must exercise **at least 30 minutes a day**. Each separate physical activity may be carried out for a relatively short time, as long as it lasts at least 10 minutes per session.

The most accessible exercise is **walking**. You should walk at a pace which allows you to have a conversation without getting out of breath. At this pace, walking is considered a moderate form activity. This kind of regular physical activity burns a lot of excess energy and helps to keep one's weight down.

6. Which forms of exercise require varied degrees of intensity (low, moderate, elevated)?

The following chart shows some examples of physical activity and indicates the level of effort usually required.

Low or very low intensity	Moderate intensity	Elevated intensity
Walking at a normal pace	Walking fast	Shovelling
Playing volley-ball	Mowing the lawn	Going to an aerobic dance course
Playing golf with a golfcart	Riding a bicycle	Jogging
Doing light gardening chores	Raking leaves	Playing hockey
Doing bowling	Playing golf without a golfcart	Playing soccer
Doing stretching exercises	Swimming	Playing basketball
Shopping	Dancing Playing tennis Downhill skiing Going to an aqua-fitness class	Cross-country skiing

7. How do people measure the difficulty level of a physical activity and progress at their own pace?

Since it is strongly recommended to start out slowly in any exercise program and increase the pace little by little, it is important to know how to measure the physical effort required. This will help you to determine your limits and measure your progress. There are two ways to evaluate your effort.

1) The degree of breathlessness: Find the level at which your breathing is heavier than when you are at rest, while at the same time you are still able to carry on a conversation without the interruptions of huffing and puffing.

2) Measure your pulse or heart rate: For an activity considered to be moderately intensite, your pulse rate should fall between 50% and 70% of your maximum level of heart beats per minute. Calculate your pulse by subtracting your age from 220 beats per minute and then multiplying the result by 50% or 70%.

For example, if a person is 45 years old:

$$(220 - 45) \times 50\% = 87.5$$

$$(220 - 45) \times 70\% = 122.5$$

To stay in a moderate activity zone, this person must keep his or her heart rate between 88 and 123 beats per minute.

8. When can exercise be dangerous for a person with diabetes?

Exercise may be hazardous or even contraindicated when diabetes is poorly controlled and blood glucose is:

1) below 4 mmol/l;

2) above 14.0 mmol/l, with the presence of ketone bodies in the urine or blood;

3)   above 17.0 mmol/l, with or without the presence of ketone bodies in the urine or blood.

In certain situations, people with diabetes may engage in regular physical activity, but they must make wise choices concerning the types of activities they take up.

Also, if:

1)   **the person with diabetes has cardiac problems,** he or she should engage in the activity while under medical supervision, with his or her doctor or health care team monitoring progress;

2)   **the person with diabetes has eye problems, with a risk of hemorrhaging,** he or she should take up physical activities such as swimming, walking and riding a stationary bike rather than anaerobic activities like weightlifting, or activities which may involve blows or jolts such as boxing, racket sports (tennis, badminton) and jogging;

3)   **the person with diabetes has serious neuropathy with complete loss of sensation in the feet,** he or she should take up activities such as swimming, biking, rowing, aerobic exercises (focussing on the arms) or exercises done while seated.

As a rule, even in the most extreme cases, walking for short periods remains one of the safest and therefore best activities.

9.   How hazardous is exercise for a person with diabetes taking oral antidiabetic medications or insulin?

A person with diabetes treated with insulin or with medications that stimulate the pancreas to produce more insulin (e.g., glyburide, gliclazide, repaglinide) is at risk for **hypoglycemia**, especially if the activity is unplanned, prolonged and moderately intensite.

Remember that:

1) **moderate exercise sustained** for several hours may cause delayed hypoglycemia, which can occur at late as 12 to 16 hours after the activity. For example, cross-country skiing, housecleaning or even shopping are all activities which may provoke delayed hypoglycemia;

2) the more **regular** the activity (schedule, duration and intensity), the lower the risk of hypoglycemia.

10. What precautions should people take when they want to engage in exercise?

1) People with diabetes should measure their blood glucose **before** engaging in any form of physical activity, regardless of their treatment regimen.

2) They should check the condition of their feet **before and after** any exercise.

3) They should not consume alcohol **before, during or after** exercise.

4) They should wear a bracelet or pendant identifying them as a person with diabetes.

If you are being treated with insulin, try to choose an injection site that you will not be using much as you exercise, for example, your abdomen.

11. What strategies can a person with diabetes taking insulin use to prevent hypoglycemia during exercise or physical activity?

A person with diabetes **being treated with rapid-or short-acting insulin** before meals should know how to adapt his or her treatment regimen in order to prevent hypoglycemia during exercise or physical activity. Let us look at the following tips.

1) When the activity is **planned, and occurs one to two hours after a meal**, reduce the insulin dose before the meal according to the type of exercise, its duration, its intensity, the training it entails and above all, according to your own experience in this regard.

   Here is a possible scenario involving exercise and decreasing insulin doses before a meal:

Example:

Intensity of effort	Percentage (%) of reduction in the rapid- or short-acting insulin dose according to duration of exercise	
	30 minutes	60 minutes
Low	25	50
Moderate	50	75
High	75	100

Suppose a person with diabetes usually injects 10 units of insulin before a meal. He or she plans on taking a moderately brisk walk, after eating, for about an hour. He or she can reduce the insulin dose by 75% and inject 2.5 units (or 3 units) before the meal:

   75% x 10 units = 7.5 units; thus,

   10 units – 7.5 units = 2.5 (or 3) units.

2) When an activity is **unplanned and occurs immediately before or after a meal**, or when the activity is **planned but occurs more than two hours after a meal**, do the following:

   ➤ **if blood glucose levels are below 5.0 mmol/l**, have a snack containing carbohydrates (15 g to 30 g) right before exercising, and, if possible, every 30 to 45 minutes thereafter during the activity;

➤ **if blood glucose levels are above 5.0 mmol/l,** have a snack with about 15 g of carbohydrates every 30 to 45 minutes during the activity.

Always measure your blood glucose immediately after exercising in order to adjust the necessary amounts of insulin and carbohydrates.

In each of these cases, the need for insulin may decrease **after exercising;** this may sometimes call for a reduction of the insulin dose taken at the following mealtime or at bedtime.

12. What strategies can a person with diabetes use to prevent hypoglycemia during exercise, if he or she is being treated with oral antidiabetic medications that stimulate the secretion of insulin?

For people with diabetes taking **medications that stimulate the pancreas to produce insulin (e.g., glyburide, gliclazide, repaglinide),** the only way to lower the risk of hypoglycemia is to consume more carbohydrates. A person with diabetes is therefore advised to do the following:

➤ **if blood glucose levels are below 5.0 mmol/l,** have a snack containing carbohydrates (15 g to 30 g) at the beginning of exercise, and, if needed, every 30 to 45 minutes thereafter during the activity;

➤ **if blood glucose levels are above 5.0 mmol/l,** additional carbohydrates are only necessary if the hypoglycemia occurs during the exercise. It is vital to know what the glycemic reading is before eating, in order to avoid overconsumption. If additional carbohydrates are necessary, have a snack with about 15 g of carbohydrates after every 30 to 45 minutes of the activity.

The following chart may serve as a guide for adding carbohydrates during physical activity. Adding carbohydrates is especially useful for unplanned exercise and is almost always necessary when exercising for extended periods of time or when doing high-intensity forms of exercise.

Type of exercise	Blood glucose (mmol/l)	Additional carbohydrates
Short duration (< 30 min.) light intensity	< 5.0	10 g to 15 g
	> 5.0	not necessary
Moderate duration (30 min. to 60 min.) moderate intensity	< 5.0	30 g to 45 g
	5.0-9.9	15 g every 30 min. to 45 min. of exercice
	10.0-13.9	not necessary
Long duration (> 60 min.) high intensity	< 5.0	45 g
	5.0-9.9	30 g to 45 g
	> 9.9	15 g per hour

13. What precautions should be taken by a person with diabetes being treated with insulin or taking oral antidiabetic medications that stimulate the secretion of insulin?

When a person with diabetes is being treated with insulin or is taking oral antidiabetic medications that stimulate the secretion of insulin, he or she must:

1) always measure blood glucose before, during and after a session of exercise. It is important to be particularly careful and, therefore, to measure blood glucose levels even more often than usual during the 24 hours that follow lengthy period of exercise session.

2) always keep on hand foods containing carbohydrates, in order to correct hypoglycemia.

CHAPTER 21

Hyperglycemic Emergencies:

Diabetic Acidosis and the Hyperosmolar State

1. What hyperglycemic emergencies can affect a person with diabetes?

Two hyperglycemic emergencies can affect a person with diabetes they are:

➤ diabetic acidosis;

➤ hyperosmolar states.

These two conditions are caused by a lack of insulin. Episodes of diabetic acidosis are more common in people with type 1 diabetes, while people with type 2 diabetes, usually when they are older, are more at risk of developing a hyperosmolar state. However, both conditions can occur simultaneously in either type 1 or type 2 diabetes.

2. What is diabetic acidosis?

Diabetic acidosis, which is attributable to insulin shortage in the body, is characterized by hyperglycemia and an accumulation of ketone bodies in the blood. The blood becomes acidic and as a result, the individual may experience **excessive fatigue, abdominal pains, nausea** and **vomiting**. Diabetic acidosis gives the breath a fruity odour, causes intense thirst, deep and rapid breathing, and occasionally makes a person feel disoriented and confused. This serious condition can sometimes result in a **coma**, which may be fatal if it is not treated.

Diabetic acidosis occurs mostly in people with type 1 diabetes, but it can occur in people with type 2 diabetes when there are other aggravating factors such as infection, myocardial infarction, pancreatitis or stroke.

3.   What causes diabetic acidosis?

Diabetic acidosis is **always** caused by a **lack of insulin** in the blood. When insulin is lacking, glucose cannot enter certain cells of the body, and this causes the glucose to accumulate in the blood at extremely high levels. The body must then draw on its reserves of fat for energy. The **breakdown of fats** produces ketone bodies, which are acidic, and they in turn accumulate in the blood and spill over into the urine.

Diabetic acidosis is a complication of diabetes, which can occur if a person **forgets** or **skips his or her insulin injections**, or **miscalculates their dosage**.

Diabetic acidosis is sometimes caused by an **increased need for insulin** (this may happen, for example, when a person gets an infection or is under exceptional stress).

4.   How can diabetic acidosis be detected?

Diabetic acidosis can be detected by the **presence of ketone bodies** in the urine or blood; these are accompanied by elevated blood glucose levels, often **higher than 20 mmol/l**.

5. How can diabetic acidosis be avoided?

Diabetic acidosis can be avoided in most cases by taking the following precautions:

1) **Check your blood glucose regularly.** You can also check for the presence of ketone bodies in the urine by using Ketostix® test strips or determine the level of ketone bodies in the blood by using the Precision Xtra® meter using a blood sample from your fingertip. **Take these readings more frequently** when you are ill, under exceptional stress, and especially if your blood glucose reading is **higher than 14 mmol/l.**

2) **Follow the meal plan recommended** by your dietician.

3) **Take insulin doses** as prescribed.

4) **Follow the advice and instructions** of your doctor and dietician concerning diet, both solid and liquid. You may add extra insulin using a sliding scale provided by your doctor when special circumstances such as illness make it difficult or impossible to follow your normal diet.

5) **Call your doctor or go to the emergency department in any one of the following five situations:**

   ➤ **your blood glucose level is above 20 mmol/l;**

   ➤ the reading of **ketone bodies in the urine is moderate (4 mmol/l) or high (8 mmol/l – 16 mmol/l);**

   ➤ the reading of **ketone bodies (ketosis level) from the fingertip is above 3 mmol/l;**

   ➤ **you are vomiting continually and cannot retain liquids;**

   ➤ the **following conditions persist** despite treatment: excessive fatigue, weakness, dizziness, abdominal pains, nausea and vomiting, fruity breath, intense thirst, fast and heavy breathing.

6.   What is a hyperosmolar state?

A hyperosmolar state usually occurs in a person with type 2 diabetes who develops a resistance to insulin. Because of this **insulin resistance, glucose** does not enter the cells well, and thus **accumulates in the blood**.

If kidney function is slightly impaired, it becomes more difficult to eliminate the excess sugar in the blood through the urine. Therefore, sugar can accumulate in the blood until it reaches very high levels (**above 30 mmol/l**), especially if the person is not drinking enough fluids. However, the small amount of insulin present in the blood at this point is sufficient to prevent the breakdown of fats, and generally diabetic acidosis does not develop.

What often happens in the case of a hyperosmolar state is that the blood glucose level rises and the person feels extremely tired and thirsty (although some elderly people feel no thirst); another symptom is frequent and profuse urination, which can lead to dehydration. This may be followed by a drop in blood pressure and, occasionally, a decrease in mental alertness that may progress to stupor, coma and sometimes death, if left untreated.

7.   What causes a hyperosmolar state?

A hyperosmolar state is always caused by a **lack of insulin** in the blood.

This is a complication of diabetes, which may occur if the person **forgets** or **skips** their insulin doses and antidiabetic medications.

A hyperosmolar state is sometimes caused by an **increased need for insulin** (for example, in case of illness, infection, exceptional stress or when the subject is using certain medications such as cortisone).

Most of the time, a hyperosmolar state occurs in people who do not **feel thirst** or who cannot hydrate themselves (drink fluids). It sometimes develops in elderly people or in individuals who cannot look after themselves adequately due to illness.

8. How can a hyperosmolar state be detected?

The symptoms of a hyperosmolar state are **intense thirst, frequent** and **increased urination** over several days, and, above all, **blood glucose levels over 30 mmol/l.** In a hyperosmolar state, there is usually no accumulation of ketone bodies in the blood or urine.

9. How can a hyperosmolar state be avoided?

The following advice can generally help you avoid a hyperosmolar state.

1) **Keep yourself hydrated**; drink 250 ml of water every hour if blood glucose levels are high or if these abnormally high values result in an increased amount and frequency of urination.

2) **Check your blood glucose level regularly** during illness or when you are under exceptional stress.

3) **Follow the meal plan** recommended by your dietician.

4) Take **antidiabetic medications** as prescribed.

5) **Follow the recommendations** of your doctor and dietician concerning **diet** (solid food and liquids) and the specially prescribed **doses of antidiabetic medications** that are to be taken when illness makes it impossible for you to follow your normal diet.

SUMMARY

Appropriate, action is determined on the basis of:

1) blood glucose levels;

2) the presence or absence of ketone bodies in urine or blood;

3) the presence of signs and symptoms.

SUGGESTED APPROACH FOR DETECTION AND TREATMENT OF DIABETIC KETOACIDOSIS AND/OR HYPEROSMOLAR STATES			
Blood glucose (mmol/l)	**Ketone bodies (mmol/l) in urine or blood**	**Symptoms**	**Suggested actions**
13–14	None, or trace Urine: 0.5 Blood: less than 0.6	Frequent urination Intense thirst	• Drink 250 ml of water every 6 hours. • Check blood glucose every 6 hours.
14–20	Low Urine: 1.5 Blood: 0.6 to 1.5	Frequent urination Intense thirst	• Drink 250 ml of water every hour. • Measure blood glucose and ketone bodies within 4 hours. • Adjust insulin doses according to the **rules of adjustment**. • Contact your doctor.
14–20	Moderate Urine: 4 Blood: 1.5 to 3	Frequent urination Intense thirst Nausea Vomiting	• Measure blood glucose and ketone bodies within 4 hours. • **Immediately** adjust the insulin dose according to **recommendations for sick days** (see boxed insert on the next page). • Contact your doctor or go to the hospital if there is no improvement.
More than 20	Moderate to high Urine: 8 to 13 Blood: more than 3 Fruity breath	Abdominal pain Nausea Vomiting	• Go to the hospital*.
More than 30	None or low Urine: 0 to 1.5 Blood: 0 to 0.6	Frequent urination Intense thirst Extreme weakne	• Go to the hospital**.

* This is an episod of diabetic acidosis.
** This is a hyperosmolar state.

Sliding scale for ajusting insulin doses on sick days : As an example, one unit of rapid- or short-acting insulin could be added for each mmol/l above a blood glucose level of 14 mmol/l, before each meal, at bedtime or, if necessary, even at night.

CHAPTER 22

Chronic Complications

1. What are the long-term complications associated with diabetes?

After a period of several years, if blood glucose levels have been elevated most of the time, complications can develop that affect:

1) the **eyes**;

2) the **kidneys**;

3) the **nervous system**; and

4) the **heart** and **blood vessels**.

2. How can diabetes affect the eyes?

Over time, hyperglycemia can cause **changes in the small blood vessels in the back of the eye (the retina)**, that may compromise blood circulation and result in haemorrhage: this is called diabetic retinopathy. If retinopathy is not adequately treated, it can lead to blindness.

3. How can you find out if your eyes have been affected by diabetes?

If your eyes are affected, you may see **spiderwebs** or **spots** in your field of vision. Contact an ophthalmologist, that is, a physician who is a specialist in eye diseases, or an optometrist.

However, changes in your eyes most often occur without impairing your vision. This highlights the **importance of seing an ophthalmologist or an optometrist regularly.**

In the case of type 1 diabetes, consult an ophthalmologist or optometrist five years after the initial diagnosis, and annually thereafter. In the case of type 2 diabetes, see an ophthalmologist or optometrist the moment you are diagnosed, and annually after that. However, in the cases of both type 1 and type 2 diabetes, if your eyes show signs of being affected, it may be necessary to see an ophthalmologist more often.

Temporary changes in sight (blurred vision) can be throught on by changes in your blood sugar levels. **Hyperglycemia and hypoglycemia can cause blurred vision**; this is corrected by normalizing your blood glucose levels.

4.   How can you protect your eyes?

To protect your eyes:

1)   keep your **blood glucose levels** as close to normal as possible;

2)   see an **ophthalmologist** or optometrist regularly;

3)   control your **blood pressure**;

4)   **quit smoking**, if applicable.

5.   What long-term effects can diabetes have on the kidneys?

In the long term, hyperglycemia can cause changes in the **small blood vessels of the kidneys**, that compromise their filtration and purification functions: this is called **diabetic nephropathy**. If diabetes is not properly controlled, this condition can eventually develop into a complete loss of renal function. When this happens the person must then be treated by dialysis (artificial kidney) or undergo a kidney transplant.

6. How can you find out if your kidneys have been affected by diabetes?

The only way to find out if your kidneys are affected is by testing for the presence of **microalbuminuria** (small amounts of albumin in the urine). A rise in blood pressure can also signal the onset of damage to the kidneys.

7. How can you protect your kidneys?

To protect your kidneys:

1) keep your **blood glucose level** as close to normal as possible;

2) check for **albumin** in urine once a year;

3) check your **blood pressure** regularly and, if it is high, take all necessary measures to control it (that is, have it measured in conjunction with other risk factors such as blood sugar, cholesterol, etc.).

4) **quit smoking**, if applicable.

8. What long-term effects can diabetes have on your nerves?

In the long term, hyperglycemia can cause **damage to the nerves**, especially in the extremities, but also to such organs as the intestines, the stomach, the bladder, the heart and the genitals. This is a condition known as **diabetic neuropathy**.

9. How can you find out whether the nerves in your extremities have been affected by diabetes?

If you notice a **decrease in the sensitivity of your extremities to pain, heat and cold, it could be a sign of nerve damage.** Another symptom is feeling a tingling or a burning sensation. The diagnosis can be confirmed by your doctor or by a special test called an electromyography (EMG).

10. When nerves in the extremities have been affected, what is the biggest danger?

The biggest danger involved in a decrease in sensation, especially in the feet, is **hurting yourself** (by wearing tight shoes, burning yourself with hot water, pricking yourself with a needle, etc.) **without noticing it**; an injury of this sort can become infected and, if circulation is compromised, can lead to gangrene and amputation.

11. How can you find out if the nerves of the intestines have been affected by diabetes?

When the nerves of the intestines are affected by diabetes, bowel movements may become difficult: this is commonly known as **constipation**. In an advanced state, when stools stagnate in the colon, the normal bacteria living in the intestines can multiply, liquefying the stools and triggering sudden and heavy diarrhea several times a day, especially at night: this is called **diabetic diarrhea**.

Constipation can first be treated through diet. A good way to counteract the condition is to gradually increase your fibre consumption and drink plenty of water. Fibre supplements in capsules or powder (e.g., Metamucil®) can help pass stools and make them firmer. If fibre and water are of no use, you can treat constipation with medication.

Constipation can be treated with medications that contract the intestines (e.g., domperidone or metoclopramide). Laxatives can also be used, such as docusate sodium or sennosides.

Diabetic diarrhea can be treated with antibiotics such as tetracycline or erythromycin. Sometimes, you must add anti-diarrheal agents such as loperamide or diphenoxylate to help alleviate the problem.

12. How can you find out if the nerves in the stomach have been affected by diabetes?

When the nerves in the stomach have been affected, the stomach empties more slowly: this is known as **diabetic gastroparesis**. Regurgitation and/or sensation of bloating after a meal is often an indication of diabetic gastroparesis. With this condition, food absorption becomes irregular, which may explain the onset of poor blood glucose control (hyperglycemia and hypoglycemia). A diagnosis can be confirmed by a nuclear medicine test of gastric emptying.

Gastroparesis can be treated with small and frequent meals and medications that contract the stomach such as domperidone or metoclopramide, as needed.

13. How can you find out if the nerves in the bladder have been affected by diabetes?

When the nerves in the bladder have been affected by diabetes, you can no longer feel when your bladder is full; also, during urination, the bladder will not empty completely: this is referred to as **neurogenic bladder**. This condition may cause a trickling overflow of urine and, if urine stagnates in the bladder, there is a risk of urinary tract infection that can extend to the kidneys.

Neurogenic bladder can be diagnosed with an echography of the bladder after urination, which will reveal any urine retention.

To avoid any overflow of urine, you should urinate regularly and thereby exert healthy pressure on your bladder. If there is considerable urine retention, your doctor can prescribe medication that will contract the bladder, such as bethanechol.

14. How can you find out if the nerves in the heart have been affected by diabetes?

Usually, even if the nerves in the heart have been affected, the condition may be asymptomatic. You can sometimes notice an accelerated heartbeat (tachycardia) and/or arrhythmia. Your doctor can help to confirm the diagnosis by prescribing an electrocardiogram (ECG).

There is no specific treatment for damaged heart nerves. If an accelerated heartbeat persists, your doctor may prescribe beta-blockers such as metoprolol, atenolol, etc.

15. How can a man find out if the nerves in his genitals have been affected by diabetes?

When the nerves in his genitals have been affected, a man with diabetes will have difficulty achieving and maintaining an erection, thus making sexual relations difficult or impossible. This condition is known as **erectile dysfunction**.

Erectile dysfunction can be treated with certain oral medications such as Viagra®, Cialis® and Levitra®. Sometimes, however, it may be necessary to use more aggressive treatments such as prostaglandin suppositories (e.g., Muse®), which are introduced into the urethra (urinary tract), or injections into the base of the penis (e.g., Caverject®).

16. Is it possible to prevent nerve problems and the complications related to them?

Yes. To prevent nerve problems and related complications, you should:

1) keep your **blood glucose level** as close to normal as possible;

2) take measures to avoid **trauma** and **burns to the feet**;

3) **inspect your feet** daily;

4) see your **doctor** if you have even the slightest lesion;

5) report any **digestive problems**;

6) report any **bladder problem**;

7) report any instances of **erectile dysfunction**;

8) report any **accelerated or irregular heartbeat**;

9) seek aggressive treatment for high**blood pressure**.

17. How can diabetes affect the heart and blood vessels?

Diabetes can affect the heart and blood vessels by accelerating the process of **arteriosclerosis**. Arteriosclerosis is a thickening and hardening of the arteries that can result in blockage of the circulation in certain parts of the body, such as the heart, the lower limbs or even the brain.

18. What are the possible dangers of this degenerative process on the heart and blood vessels?

The dangers of arteriosclerosis depend on the part of the body that is affected:

1) if the heart is affected, it can result in a **myocardial infarction**;

2) if the brain is affected, it can result in a **paralysis** (stroke);

3) if the lower limbs are affected, it can result in **painful walking** and **limping**.

19. How can you find out if the heart and blood vessels have been affected by diabetes?

Certain signs may indicate the presence of arteriosclerosis and circulatory problems:

1) **slow healing** of wounds;

2) **chest pain** and/or **difficulty breathing** during physical exertion;

3) **pain in the calves** when walking, or limping.

However, there are sometimes no symptoms associated with arteriosclerosis, especially in its early stages. In this case, it can only be diagnosed by medical examination or special tests such as an electrocardiogram (at rest or during exertion), a cardiac scintigraphy (MIBI), an abdominal X-ray (to search for vessel calcification) and, finally, a Doppler test (which is an examination of the condition of blood vessels in the neck or the lower limbs by using ultrasonography).

20. How can you prevent your heart and blood vessels from being affected by diabetes?

To reduce the risk of your heart and blood vessels being affected:

1)   keep your **blood glucose level** as close to normal as possible;

2)   have your **blood pressure** checked regularly and treat any hypertensive condition aggressively;

3)   whenever possible, avoid consuming **saturated fats** (especially of animal origin);

4)   have your **blood lipid level** checked regularly and proactively treat any anomalies observed;

5)   **quit smoking**, if applicable;

6)   **exercise regularly**;

7)   take an **aspirin a day** (unless contraindicated).

21. What is high blood pressure?

For most people, blood pressure is considered high if it is greater than or equal to 140/90. However, for people with diabetes, the threshold is lower, so a blood pressure greater than or equal to 130/80 is considered high for them.

22. Why should hypertension be treated aggressively in a person with diabetes?

Hypertension considerably increases the risk of diabetes-related complications that can affect the eyes, nerves, kidneys, heart and blood vessels.

It has been proven that treating hypertension in people with diabetes significantly decreases the appearance and progression of complications associated with the disease.

23. What is considered an abnormal blood lipid in a person with diabetes?

A person with diabetes is said to have a blood lipid abnormality if:

1)   bad cholesterol (LDL-cholesterol) is greater than or equal to 2.5 mmol/l;

2)   good cholesterol (HDL-cholesterol) is less than or equal to 1.0 mmol/l;

3)   triglycerides are greater than or equal to 1.5 mmol/l; or

4)   the ratio between total cholesterol over HDL-cholesterol is greater than or equal to 4.0.

24.   Why should all blood lipid abnormalities be aggressively treated?

Blood lipid abnormalities should be treated aggressively because they are major risk factors for developing arteriosclerosis and related diseases of the heart and blood vessels. Since people with diabetes have a higher risk of developing these kinds of diseases to begin with, they must be treated with particular care in this regard.

CHAPTER 23

Foot Care and General Hygiene Measures

1. Why is diabetic foot care a public healthcare issue?

Diabetic foot complications are a major public healthcare issue because they are the principal cause of non-trauma-related amputations. Over a period of time, poorly controlled diabetes is associated with peripheral neuropathy, especially of the feet. Loss of sensitivity to touch, pain, heat and cold are some of the symptoms of the condition. This loss of sensitivity makes the person with diabetes vulnerable to injuries that go unnoticed. Any lesion can become infected and, if there are circulatory problems, gangrene can develop, sometimes requiring amputation. Nevertheless, if people with diabetes take good care of their feet, they can prevent 80% of these amputations. Hence the importance of learning proper foot care.

2. In people with diabetes, which problems can lead to complications related to the feet?

The feet of a person with diabetes are more fragile than those of a person that does not have the disease. In the long term, hyperglycemia can lead to the following foot problems:

1) **damage to nerves** with loss of sensitivity to touch, pain, heat and cold;

2)   a tendency for the skin to get thinner and drier, to become more easily irritated and to develop calluses (hyperkeratosis) at pressure points;

3)   a tendency for arteries to thicken and harden, thereby compromising circulation in the feet;

4)   a susceptibility to infection, because the body is less able to defend itself against microbes when blood glucose levels are high.

3.   How should you examine your feet?

A person with diabetes should share the responsibility for foot care with his or her healthcare team. In order to prevent complications, you should:

1)   examine your feet closely every day after a bath or shower;

2)   use a good light source and, when seated, examine both feet from every possible angle (from below and above; also check between the toes);

3)   use a mirror to examine the soles of your feet, if you are not flexible enough to see them without one;

4)   ask for help from a person close to you if you have impaired vision or cannot reach your feet;

5)   follow up your self-exam with a detailed professional examination each time you see a doctor or nurse specialized in foot care.

4.   What should you look for?

Look carefully for:

1)   lesions between the toes caused by fungi that thrive in humid conditions (athlete's foot);

2)   calluses: heavily callused skin (often located under the foot), should be treated appropriately, because calluses can make your skin fragile, vulnerable to infection, and as such provide a good place for microbes to multiply in;

3) corns situated:

➡ on the toes, produced by friction with shoes;

➡ between the toes, known as "soft corns" (or "kissing corns"), because the moisture existing between the toes causes them to be softer than regular hard corns. Soft corns are produced by, that are toes pressed or "squashed" against one another, thus creating a moist environment.

4) cracks: these crevices in callused skin (often on or around the heel) are particularly well-suited for microbial growth. This excess callused skin can always be traced to a specific cause:

➡ poor foot posture (position, compression); see your doctor as soon as possible;

➡ avoid using instruments that can harm the feet: razor blades, knives, graters or corn-removal preparations;

➡ foreign bodies in the shoes or seams that can injure the feet; check for them by running your hand along the inside of your shoes.

5. What are the first signs of foot problems?

You should examine your feet for:

1) changes in skin colour, unusual redness;

2) high skin temperature;

3) swollen feet or ankles;

4) pain in the legs or feet;

5) ingrown toenails;

6) toenail fungi;

7) open sores that heal slowly;

8) bleeding calluses;

9) dry and fissured skin, especially around the heel;

10) scratches;

11) bunions;

12) warts;

13) loss of sensation in the feet.

6. How can a person with diabetes reduce the risk of foot problems?

To limit the risk of developing foot problems:

1) keep blood glucose level as close to normal as possible;

2) quit smoking, if applicable;

3) lose weight, if necessary;

4) reduce your alcohol consumption, if applicable;

5) get regular exercise;

6) see a doctor, podiatrist, or nurse specialized in foot care or any other specialist as needed.

7. What are the 10 suggestions of foot care for people with diabetes?

1) **Examine your feet every day** and ask for help from family and friends, as needed:

➤ examine your feet closely all over, looking for lesions, cuts, bruises or any other changes;

➤ regularly check the sensitivity level of your feet (according to your doctor's recommendations):

• run a cotton ball lightly over and under your foot to detect any areas lacking sensation;

- put an dry pea in your shoe and walk a few steps to see if you can detect the presence of a foreign body; remove the pea to avoid injuring yourself.

2) **Do not walk barefoot, not even in the house,** and especially not on a beach or in any public area:

➡ wear slippers if you get up during the night;

➡ wear comfortable shoes.

3) **Wash your feet every day:**

➡ check the water temperature with your wrist, elbow or with a thermometer; the water should be lukewarm (below 37°C);

➡ wash your feet with a mild soap (e.g., Dove® unscented, Aveeno®, Cetaphil®, Neutrogena®, Keri®, etc.);

➡ do not soak your feet for more than 10 minutes to avoid maceration and softening of the skin;

➡ dry your feet carefully, especially between and under the toes; humidity favours the development of fungi such as athlete's foot.

4) **Check if the skin is very dry:**

➡ apply a neutral (unscented) moisturizing cream (e.g., Nivea®, Lubriderm®, Vaseline Intensive Care® (Lotion), Glycerodermine®, etc.) in a thin layer, except between the toes;

➡ use a moistened pumice stone to rub areas where hyperkeratosis (thickening of the skin) has developed after a bath or shower, once or twice a week; use continual rather than back and forth movements; use of a metal grater is strongly discouraged.

5) **Keep your nails sufficiently long:**

➡ keep your nails square and a little longer than the end of your toes (do that after a bath or a shower); this will keep ingrown toenails and wounds from developing;

➡ file down nails rather than cutting them; an emery board helps to avoid injuries;

➡ handle round-ended scissors and nailclippers with care; avoid using them if you are not dexterous, or have impaired or reduced vision;

➡ never rip or tear nails.

6)   Never treat calluses, corns or blisters yourself:

➡ do not perform "bathroom surgery;" never use pointy scissors, clippers, razor blades, lancets or scalpels, or metal files to remove a corn;

➡ never use solutions or plasters with a salicylic acid base (these are available over the counter in pharmacies); they can cause necrosis of skin tissue;

➡ see a professional who specialist in foot care; inform him or her that you have diabetes.

7)   Change your socks every day:

➡ wear clean socks (or stockings); wash them every day;

➡ wear socks that are the right size; make sure they are loose and long enough to avoid squeezing the toes; avoid wearing tight socks that leave marks on the calves and cut off circulation;

➡ avoid thick stitching; if socks have seams, wear them inside out;

➡ avoid shoes with holes or patches that may cause points of friction;

➡ choose socks that keep the feet dry, made from a blend of cotton and synthetic fibres (acrylic, orlon, polypropylene, coolmax, etc.); people who sweat profusely should avoid socks containing nylon.

8)   Choose your shoes carefully:

➡ always wear socks with your shoes;

➡ choose shoes fastened with laces, buckles or velcro; they should be made from supple leather or from canvas and be big enough to allow the toes to move;

➤ choose non-skid soles no thicker than 4 cm;

➤ buy shoes in the late afternoon: when feet are swollen, it is easier to choose shoes that fit you;

➤ break in new shoes gradually; start wearing them a half-hour a day;

➤ carefully inspect the inside of shoes before wearing them; run your hand inside them to find any foreign bodies or seams which could injure your feet;

➤ avoid pointy shoes and those with high heels.

9) **Watch out for burns or frostbite:**

➤ wear socks, even in bed, if your feet are cold; avoid hot-water bottles, electric blankets or hot water;

➤ use sunscreen with an SPF (sun protection factor) of at least 15 to lower the risk of sunstroke;

➤ never use powerful products or irritants (e.g., Parisienne® or other bleaches);

➤ make sure skin is covered, especially in winter, when the weather is cold and dry.

10) **Immediately contact** your footcare specialist (doctor, podiatrist or nurse) if you notice discolouration, loss of sensation or a lesion.

8. What moisturizing creams can a person with diabetes use for foot care?

When a person's skin has a tendency to dry out, the daily use of a moisturizer is recommended. Use unscented products without colouring and with a neutral pH. Avoid applying cream between the toes, to prevent over softening skin. Apply a fine layer after a bath or shower.

There are three main kinds of moisturizing products:

1) **hydrating products with humectants,** which soften the skin and diminish fine lines (e.g., Nivea®, Glycerodermine®, Glaxal Base®, Aquatain®, Complex-15®, etc.);

2) **anti-dehydration products,** which reduce the evaporation of moisture by forming a film on the skin (e.g., Moisturel®, Lubriderm® (Lotion), Cetaphil®, Aveeno® (Lotion), Keri® (Lotion), Vaseline Intensive Care® (Lotion), Neutrogena®, Aquaphor®, Prevez®, Barrier Creme®, Akildia®, Curel®, Eucrin®, Elta®, etc.);

3) **hydrating products with keratolytic and exfoliating properties,** which help remove dead skin cells. These products should be used with caution, and be applied on the stratum corneum or top layer of the skin. Urea may cause a burning or tingling sensation on dry or cracked skin (e.g., Uremol-10®, Uremol-20®, Dermal Therapy 25% urea, Lacticare® (Lotion), Lac-Hydrin® (Lotion), Urisec®, etc.).

9. Which antiseptic products can a person with diabetes use for sores or wounds on the feet?

There are several available products that are helpful. Before applying any of them, wash the wound with water and mild soap, then rinse and dry it well. Next, follow these steps and recommendations:

1) **Disinfect the skin with an antiseptic** (according to a doctor's recommendations):

➤ 70% alcohol swab;

➤ proviodine swab;

➤ Hibidil® (chlorhexidine gluconate 0.05%);

➤ Baxedin®;

➤ Steristat®.

2) **If there is inflammation**, apply a compress soaked in physiological saline solution three or four times a day. Watch for signs of infection during the next 24 to 48 hours. Avoid using adhesive tape directly on the skin. If redness worsens or if then is pus, see a doctor immediately.

3) In case your doctor recommends foot baths, use one of the following products in a litre of lukewarm boiled water for no more than 10 minutes:

➤ 15 ml (1 tbsp.) of Proviodine®;

➤ 15 ml (1 tbsp.) of Hibitane® 4% (chlorhexidine gluconate 4%) ;

➤ 30 ml (2 tbsp.) of Hibitane® 2% (chlorhexidine gluconate 2%).

Wash your feet again in running water and dry them well, especially between the toes. See a doctor if the sore does not mend.

It is important to discover the cause of the problem so that it is does not come back.

10. How can you improve the circulation in your feet?

There are a number of simple methods available to all that can improve circulation and maintain or improve the flexibility of the feet.

➤ Avoid smoking.

➤ Uncross your legs when seated.

➤ Keep moving – do not remain standing or seated in one place for too long.

➤ Walk as much as you can, within your limits and abilities.

➤ When seated, rest your legs on a footstool whenever possible.

➤ Do foot exercises regularly – repeat each one 20 times:

- put a towel on the floor and try to pick it up with your toes;

- stand on the tips of your toes; then lower your body weight down onto your heels; use a support if necessary (be careful not to fall);

- point your feet up and down by flexing your ankle;

- rotate your feet, first in one direction, then the other;

- rock yourself in an armchair, pushing yourself with your toes.

11. What is a diabetic foot ulcer?

A diabetic foot ulcer is an example of a foot wound resulting from neuropathy; it develops on pressure points under the foot, due to calluses and other foot deformations. Because a person with diabetes often lacks sensitivity in his or her feet, he or she often continues to walk on the wound, unwittingly making it worse. At this stage, a sore may appear in the middle of the callus. The wound can worsen even and become infected, especially if blood glucose is poorly controlled; if the sore is not treated adequately, it can become gangrenous and amputation may then be necessary.

If you have any questions about the nature of a wound, see your doctor as quickly as possible, since a foot ulcer can be healed with appropriate treatment.

12. Why should a person with diabetes practice dental hygiene?

As in the case of skin or feet, you should manage your dental health with special care for two major reasons:

1)   There is a high risk of cavities, gum sores or infection if diabetes is poorly controlled.

2)   Any infection can raise blood glucose levels and hamper control of diabetes.

Therefore, brushing and flossing your teeth are essential.

See a dentist once or twice a year, according to your personal health condition.

See a denturist every five years for adjustment of any dental prostheses, if applicable.

CHAPTER 24

Living With Diabetes

1. What does living with diabetes mean?

Despite the fact that diabetes is becoming more and more widespread, many people find that **it is not easy to live with the disease**.

Being diagnosed with the disease poses a series of challenges that a person with diabetes must face for the rest of his or her life. Here are a few of those challenges.

1) **Realizing that diabetes is a chronic illness** that cannot be cured.

2) **Acknowledging that diabetes is a serious illness**, even if the early symptoms are hardly noticeable or painful.

3) **Accepting the necessity of establishps a daily routine** (meals, sleep, exercise, etc.), especially if the person is being treated with insulin.

4) **Motivating oneself to make lifestyle changes**, because medication alone is not enough to treat diabetes.

5) **Taking personal responsibility** for the treatment.

The challenges of diabetes are considerable, but by no means insurmountable.

2.   What can be of help to a person who has just learned that he or she has diabetes?

First of all, there is good news, and there are plenty of reasons to feel hopeful. The evolution of the medical and psychosocial understanding of diabetes allows people with the disease to be optimistic. As silver linings are continually being discovered in the clouds of diabetes research, we should realize that:

1)   diabetes is a disease which **can be controlled effectively**;

2)   good control of blood glucose **significantly decreases the risks of developing serious complications** down the road;

3)   the availability of information and training resources, such as diabetes seminars, allows people with diabetes to acquire the necessary skills **to adapt their treatment to the changes of daily life and individual needs**;

4)   diabetes can be an **opportunity to learn** how to improve diet, to take up regular exercise, to better manage stress, and thus to learn how to live better.

It is therefore possible for the majority of people with diabetes to live long, active, prosperous, healthy and satisfying lives.

3.   How can a person with diabetes learn to accept and cope with the reality that he or she has the disease?

When diagnosed with diabetes, a person will go through a period of emotional shock even though he or she might not be aware of it. This shock is caused by having to deal with the loss inevitably linked to the reality of having a chronic disease.

Whether he or she wants it or not, the emotional shock triggers a grieving process. It is this grieving process that will lead the person, at his or her own speed, to a state of acceptance of the disease and, ultimately, of its treatment.

The grieving process is assuaged and becomes much easier to deal with if one has a better understanding of the disease. It is therefore important to find out about diabetes; a greater understanding of the disease can help you to better accept it.

4.   What is a grieving process?

A grieving process is a process of emotional growth that all people must go through when dealing with a loss. In the case of diabetes, this principally involves grieving the loss of one's health; however, it also means coming to terms with some other equally important losses, such as the loss of a certain amount of freedom, of some spontaneity, of some old habits, and perhaps even of a feeling of invincibility.

This grieving process comprises a number of stages, which correspond to emotions of varying intensity and duration. These emotions that the person with diabetes will experience will help him or her to develop a new found emotional stability and to achieve a degree of acceptance.

5.   What are the stages of grief?

The following chart shows the five stages of grief. The order in which they occur may vary, depending on the individual.

Stage	Description	Testimonials
1) Denial or negation	Ignoring the unbearable aspects of the disease or of treatment. Acting as though you are not ill, or as though the disease is not serious.	"I cannot be have diabetes, I do not feel sick."
2) Anger or revolt	Seeing the disease as an injustice. Being "angry at the world." Blaming others. Only seeing the negative aspects of treatment.	"Diabetes is the worst disease possible, and it is preventing me from doing what I want."
3) Negotiating or bargaining	Having a tendancy to take on what suits you and to leave out whatever does not. Acceptance remains very conditional.	"I take pills to lower the sugar in my blood, so I do not have to pay attention to what I eat"
4) Depressive feelings, or reflection	Realizing that denying the disease is useless. Exaggerated perception of the limitations that come with diabetes. Possible feelings of powerlessness, helplessness, or a retreat into dependency.	"Is this kind of life worth living?"
5) Acceptance	Realistic perception of the disease and its treatment. Deciding to take concrete and positive action.	"I would rather not have diabetes, but since I do not have a choice, I am going to do my best."

6. How can you positively influence the grieving process and thereby encourage your acceptance of the disease?

First of all, having a proactive attitude towards learning will help you understand the stages of grief, identify its related emotions, and above all, help you to recognize yourself in these emotions. This involves a journey of self-knowledge and self-examination.

Next, learn to attribute some worth to the negative feelings you are experiencing, whether they be guilt, anger or fear. It is perfectly normal to experience negative feelings or emotions. Negative feelings are not bad in themselves, rather, they are experiences that simply "do not feel good" and, as one would expect, are not very pleasant to endure.

However, being aware of negative feelings may stimulate one's motivation to change. These feelings are often the expression of psychological pain related to specific problems. Therefore, the best way to ease this pain is to find solutions to the problems that are causing it.

In this way, you can affect the grieving process in a positive way, and thereby accelerate process of accepting your disease.

7. Are some emotional problems more common in people with diabetes?

Yes. While we know that depression and anxiety affect a good number of people in the general population, studies suggest that **depression** and **anxiety disorders** are more common among people with a chronic physical disease such as diabetes.

It is estimated that depression affects people with diabetes up to three times more often than it does those in the general population (20% compared to 5-10%). Similarly, anxiety disorders are up to six times more common (30% compared to 5%).

It is therefore important to diagnose these two psychological problems accurately, because they will have a significant influence on the control of blood glucose. The more depressed or anxious you feel, the harder it will be to control your diabetes.

8.   How can you recognize depression?

First of all, it is necessary to distinguish depressive feelings, which are normal emotions linked to the grieving process, from clinical depression, which is an illness. A depressed mood does not necessarily lead to a diagnosis of depression.

Depression **becomes an illness** when the symptoms (described below) **last several weeks** and begin to **affect your work and social life**. The symptoms are:

1) feeling depressed, sad, hopeless, discouraged, "at the end of your rope" most of the day, and almost every day;

2) loss of interest or pleasure in just about all activities;

3) loss of appetite or weight, or significant increase in appetite or weight;

4) insomnia or a need to sleep more than usual;

5) agitation (e.g., difficulty sitting still) or slowing down of psychomotor functions (e.g., slowed speech, monotone voice, long delay before answering a question, slower bodily movements);

6) lack of energy, tiredness;

7) feelings of lost dignity, self-blame, excessive or inappropriate guilt;

8) difficult in concentrating, thinking or making decisions;

9) recurring thoughts of death, suicidal impulses, wishing for death, or actual suicide attempts.

9.   What should you do if you think you are suffering from depression?

If you have experienced some or several of these symptoms for two weeks or more, you should inform your doctor so that he or she can determine whether the symptoms (e.g., weight loss, fatigue, loss of concentration) are due to your diabetes or to depression and direct you to get the help you need.

Although depressive feelings may be a normal part of the grieving process after a diagnosis of diabetes, it is important that you see your doctor if these feelings intensify and last for several weeks.

Depression is one of the most easily treated mental health problems, especially if it is promptly diagnosed. Most people who suffer from depression are treated with antidepressant medications and/or psychotherapy. The combination of these two therapeutic approaches is recognized as the most effective treatment available. The support of family, friends and other support groups is equally important.

10. How can you recognize an anxiety disorder?

An anxiety disorder is a mental health problem in which anxiety is the predominant disturbance. In people with diabetes, anxiety disorders such as phobias (e.g., fear of needles, fear of having low blood glucose levels) are common. **Generalized anxiety disorder (GAD)** is the most frequent disorder in this group.

A diagnosis of generalized anxiety disorder (GAD) may be made if the following symptoms appear:

1) anxiety and excessive worry most of the time, for at least six months, concerning various events or activities;

2) difficulty controlling this preoccupation;

3) intense distress;

4) agitation or feeling on edge;

5) becoming tired easily;

6) difficulty concentrating or memory lapses;

7) irritability;

8) muscular tension;

9) disturbed sleep.

11. What should you do if you think you are suffering from an anxiety disorder?

If you show signs of generalized anxiety disorder (GAD) or phobia, speak to your doctor, who will evaluate your situation and recommend appropriate treatment or, if suitable, refer you to a mental health professional.

Anxiety disorders can be treated with medication and/or psychotherapy. Relaxation techniques are often used as therapeutic tools for these conditions.

12. Where can you find help if you are suffering from depression or an anxiety disorder?

Speak to your doctor. In some cases, he or she can begin your treatment with medication, if required. He or she can also refer you to a mental health professional, such as a psychiatrist or psychologist working in the public health system. You can find these professionals at a hospital's department of psychiatry or psychology, or in mental health services offered by some local clinics.

It is also possible to see psychiatrists and psychologists in private practice. You can get in touch with these individuals by contacting their respective professional associations.

13. Is it true that the personality of a person with diabetes changes, becoming progressively angrier or more aggressive?

No. **Anger is not a personality trait particular to a person with diabetes.** There may certainly be short-tempered people with the disease in the world, but it has nothing to do with the fact that they have diabetes.

However, **a sudden change in character or mood swings characterized by irritability or anger** may be a sign that a person with diabetes is in a **hypoglycemic state**. These signs will disappear once the hypoglycemia has been corrected.

Mood swings or changes are also observed **when a person with diabetes becomes very tired** because his blood glucose level is high or fluctuating. These mood swings usually stop quickly when control of blood glucose improves and the person recovers his or her energy.

Finally, an irritable mood **may signify a lack of acceptance of the disease**. In such cases, individuals may be embittered by the disease. This phenomenon is not specific to diabetes; it can be found in any person with a chronic disease who does not accept his or her condition.

It is therefore important for the people around a person with diabetes to differentiate between the various reasons for mood swings, so as to provide some warmth, empathy and to also better understand what he or she is going through.

Remember this:

Your personality shapes your reaction to diabetes.

You cannot always control your emotions, but you are personally responsible for your behaviour.

You cannot control the time it takes to go through the grieving process, but in order to influence this process it is your responsability to become informed about diabetes and to observe your behaviour.

You are not at fault for having developed diabetes, but you are responsible for managing your disease.

CHAPTER 25

Managing Daily Stress

1. Why should a person with diabetes be concerned with daily stress?

Because stress can increase blood glucose levels in some people with diabetes. Stress can have a direct effect on blood glucose levels by promoting the release of hormones, such as adrenalin, that stimulate the liver to release glucose stored there into the bloodstream. These hormones also diminish the effect of insulin by creating a resistance of the body's cells to its action. Stress can also affect glycemia indirectly by causing people to neglect their self care.

2. Does stress cause diabetes?

No. However, stress can be a factor that triggers the disease in someone genetically predisposed to it.

3. What is stress?

Stress is what you feel when you think you cannot effectively face a situation that you perceive as being threatening.

Stress is caused by an event perceived by the individual (consciously or unconsciously) as surpassing his or her capabilities and threatening his or her well-being. This depends on two conditions:

1) the importance given to the event by the individual;

2) the imbalance between the demands coming from a person's environment, or the demands an individual places on himself or herself, and the capacity he or she has of dealing with them.

Therefore, stress is largely the result of one's perception of an event and is not necessarily related to the reality of the event itself.

Stress is a part of life. No person goes through life without encountering it. Essentially, stress is an adaptive mechanism that has allowed and will continue to allow humanity to survive. When several factors are taken into account, stress can be either good or bad.

4.   What is "good stress"?

Your capacity to effectively deal with a threatening situation is what determines whether or not you perceive stress as being good or bad. Stress can be a positive force in your life. For example, solving a very difficult problem or falling in love are both events which can cause good stress, because these situations can add to the pleasure and satisfaction you derive from life. On the other hand, if you perceive these situations as being beyond your means dealing with them in a positive manner, then you will probably experience a lot of stress and perceive it as bad stress.

5.   What are the sources of stress?

The three categories of stressors are as follows:

1)   physical stressors:

➤   illness and its consequences;

➤   fatigue;

➤   pain.

2) **psychological stressors:**

➤ emotions;

➤ attitudes;

➤ behaviour.

3) **social stressors:**

➤ interpersonal and professional relationships;

➤ death of a loved one;

➤ major life changes (marriage, moving, retirement).

It should be noted that stress can be triggered by happy events (marriage, the birth of a child, a promotion) as well as painful ones.

6. What affects our response to stress?

Several factors affect our response to stress:

1) **personal factors:** personality, past experiences, attitudes;

2) **emotions experienced when dealing with illness:** guilt, anxiety, sadness, fear, etc.;

3) **personal resources:** adaptability, support, information.

7. How can you recognize the symptoms of stress?

There are many stress indicators:

1) **physical symptoms:**

➤ increased heartbeat;

➤ rise in blood pressure;

➤ increased muscular tension;

➤ faster breathing;

> chronic fatigue;

> headaches, backache;

> tightness in the chest;

> digestive problems;

> tics, twitching.

2) **psychological symptoms:**

> aggression;

> depression;

> bouts of crying or an inability to cry;

> feelings of emptiness, dissatisfaction;

> ambivalence;

> decrease in concentration, attention;

> decreased motivation;

> loss of self-esteem;

> nightmares.

3) **behavioural symptoms:**

> irritability;

> angry outbursts;

> very critical attitude;

> forgetfulness, indecision;

> loss of productivity;

> increased consumption of some foods or substances (tobacco, alcohol, medications) or loss of appetite;

> sexual problems.

Although we can deal adequately with occasional stress, persistent, intense and frequent stress can overtax our body and create undesirable physical states. Stress is a part of human life and cannot be eliminated; but we can learn to manage and minimize its negative effects.

8. How can you respond to stress?

1) **Recognize your level of stress:** first, learn how to recognize your symptoms and sources of stress, being aware of your level of stress is a crucial starting point.

2) **Distinguish good stress and bad stress:** you must recognize what makes stress positive or negative for you.

3) **Develop strategies to adapt to stress:** research on adaptive strategies has shown that the people who adapt best, are those who use strategies focused on solving problems rather than behaviour based only on their emotional response.

9. What is a problem-solving approach?

It is a logical process that allows you to analyze a stressful situation and explore different solutions that can be applied. The steps are as follows:

1) **Step one: defining the problem.** Define the problem in simple, clear and concrete terms.

2) **Step two: researching for solutions.** Imagine as many solutions as possible without being overly self-critical.

3) **Step three: evaluating each solution considered.** Look at the advantages and disadvantages of each solution. Sort them according to the ease or difficulty of applying each one, and to your intention of implementing them.

4) **Step four: preparing a plan of action.** Decide which of the solutions you will set as your goal. Prepare a plan of action that will pinpoint the concrete actions to be performed.

10. What adaptive strategies can help to manage emotion-related stress in my everyday life?

➤ Learn how to express your negative emotions in an appropriate manner, to yourself as well as to others.

➤ Avoid belittling yourself or dramatizing the situation; try to accurately perceive the real situation.

➤ Use some positive self-affirmation to control paralyzing emotions (e.g., "I can do it", "I have made it through worse than this", "Everything is okay, this is a step in the right direction").

➤ Use relaxation techniques to lower emotional stress.

11. What adaptive strategies can I use to help manage stress related to my behaviour?

➤ Express your needs, while respecting those of others.

➤ Avoid submitting passively to events that you do not wish to participate in: do not indulge in the "martyr syndrome."

➤ Learn to say no when you truly cannot or do not want to say yes.

➤ Do not allow problems to pile up.

➤ Temporarily remove yourself from stressful situations.

12. What adaptive strategies will help you to manage stress related to your lifestyle?

➤ Plan out a balanced exercise program featuring creative and relaxing activities.

➤ Look for activities that you find fulfilling and pleasurable.

➤ Organize your time and set up realistic deadlines.

➤ Maintain some separation between your professional and personal life.

➤ Do not attempt to lower your stress by consuming excessive amounts of alcohol, food or drugs.

13. What attitudes and behaviours will help you, as a person with diabetes, manage stress related to your disease?

1) Manage your disease well:

➤ check blood glucose regularly;

➤ eat well;

➤ exercise;

➤ take your medications as prescribed;

➤ learn about diabetes.

2) Deal with external stressors:

➤ practice time management (plan, define your priorities);

➤ change your environment, if necessary;

➤ engage in satisfying activities;

➤ use relaxation techniques;

➤ avoid excessive procrastination—put things in motion as soon as possible;

➤ make changes gradually; avoid "all-or-nothing" reactions.

3)   Deal with psychological stressors:

➤   control irrational thoughts (e.g., perfectionism);

➤   question your beliefs and change them if necessary (e.g., "What I do not know cannot hurt me, so I shall think about diabetes as little as possible");

➤   open yourself up to new experiences and consider looking at life in different ways (e.g., engage in different physical activities to discover the ones that suit you best);

➤   create a varied social support network (family, friends, outreach groups) but do not overtax them (e.g., avoid making members of your family responsible for your treatment). Be sure to let them know how much you appreciate their support;

➤   talk to and share things with a person you trust: confiding in someone will help you to feel better, get things off your chest and, above all, escape from the feeling of isolation often provoked by the disease;

➤   see a specialist if your own resources seem inadequate. A psychologist is a specialist in human behaviour. He or she can help you to identify the sources of your stress, to determine your reactions to them and to change your attitudes and behaviours in order to better manage them.

14. What does relaxation involve?

Relaxation is an important tool for stress management. While stress provokes a number of reactions, stimulating several physiological functions (cardiovascular, respiratory, muscular), relaxation produces the opposite effect in these very same functions, thereby re-establishing a physiological and psychological balance. Relaxation brings more than just "rest"; its therapeutic effects are even deeper and farther reaching.

15. Are there relaxation exercises that can be done easily?

Several techniques can be used, the most common ones being:

1) active relaxation, which consists of alternatively tensing and relaxing the muscles;

2) passive relaxation, which consists of sequentially relaxing all the parts of the body, by naming each one inwardly.

The important thing is to slow down, to distance yourself from external stimuli (noise, light, activity), to sit down, to close your eyes and to breathe deeply, all at your own rhythm. You will notice that after a few minutes, your breathing will begin to slow. Next, do an inventory of all the parts of your body, starting with your feet and ending with your head. You will feel looser, more relaxed, with sensations of warmth, heaviness and calm overtaking you. With practice, five minutes will be enough to reach this state of relaxation anywhere, including public places. It is just a matter of training yourself; it is easy, it can be done by anyone and, above all, it is very effective!

16. Are there tools that promote relaxation?

A wide variety of audio cassettes provide information on relaxation techniques. Experiment and discover what you prefer.

There are some suggestions for beginners:

➤ *Progressive Relaxation and Breathing.* 1987. Oakland, CA: New Harbinger Publications Inc. Jacobson's complete Deep Muscle technique, shorthand relaxation of muscle groups, deep breathing, etc.

➤ *Applied Relaxation Training.* 1991. Oakland, CA: New Harbinger Publication Inc. How to relax all your muscles except those you actually need for a given activity, so that you can reduce your stress while driving, doing desk work or walking.

You can find a variety of books on relaxation:

➤ You will surely find interesting books at the library. It is up to you to choose. We particularly recommend *The Relaxation and Stress Reduction Workbook*, 4th edition, by Martha Davis et al., published by New Harbinger Publications.

17. Should I talk about the disease with my family and friends?

You must to realize that your family and friends will share your feelings of shock, especially when the disease is first diagnosed. It is important to speak with them. They are worried about you, and they need information in order to properly help you. Communication is always a winning formula, and you have a formative role to play. You should provide your family and friends with general information on diabetes, your lifestyle regimen, and the complications that could occur, so that you help yourself by building the finest assistance and support network possible. Expressing your needs and expectations is a good step towards coming to a mutual understanding with your family and friends; it also provides you with a measure of safety.

18. What reactions can I expect from my family and friends?

In most cases, family and friends try to help, but they do not always do it in the right fashion. Sometimes, you may have the impression that all they want to do is tell you what you should and should not do or, conversely, that they minimize the seriousness of the illness and lure you away from "the right path." Lack of information and education is usually the primary source of these dilemmas. It is therefore important to keep your family and friends informed of your needs and expectations. You are an independent person in control of your own life.

19. Should I talk about my condition at work?

It is important to find allies. In an emergency, these people can help you. It is your responsibility to create a safe environment for yourself at work. Your success or failure in bringing about changes like this, will either provoke new stresses or, on the contrary, alleviate your stress level and help you achieve a sense of well being.

CHAPTER 26

The Motivation to Change

1. What is motivation?

Motivation is the effect of conscious and unconscious forces that determine behaviour.

For example, smoking is a behaviour determined and conditioned by all kinds of motivating forces such as its relaxing effect, advertising, fashion and emotional conflicts.

You can become partly aware of these forces by analyzing the reasons you give yourself for keeping or changing a behaviour.

2. Why is motivation important in the treatment of diabetes?

First and foremost, because diabetes is a disease that requires of people that they take care of themselves (self-care) and control their own blood glucose levels (self-monitoring).

Self-care and self-monitoring will work only if the individual is willing to make changes in his or her lifestyle—choosing to eat better, exercising and managing stress.

The treatment of diabetes calls for a high degree of personal motivation to adopt or maintain behaviour favourable to good health.

3.   What are the main factors that affect the motivation to change?

There are three principal factors:

1)   The will to change

The will to change is determined in good measure by your beliefs concerning health, diabetes and its treatment.

The set of convictions called "health beliefs" has been proven to encourage the adoption of healthy behaviours (e.g., believing that the proposed treatment regimen is effective).

On the other hand, there are also false beliefs or myths – personal misconceptions regarding the disease and its treatment that can negatively affect the will to change.

2)   The steps towards change

Any transformative process is accomplished step by step. These steps can be defined by the feeling that you are more or less ready to take action. Each of these steps includes recommended actions that will accelerate your progress and help you take your "road to change" to the next level.

3)   The capacity to change

The capacity to change requires that you learn skills that encourage change.

Two of these required skills are the manner in which you set your goals, and your knowledge of the plan or strategy for change.

4.   How can the health beliefs of a person with diabetes reinforce the will to change?

Health beliefs are a set of beliefs that a person holds regarding diabetes and its treatment. They can play a positive role in reinforcing the will to change a behaviour.

The more closely you adhere to your health beliefs, the stronger will be your will to adopt behaviours that favour good health (eating better, checking blood glucose regularly, etc.). To evaluate the sincerity of your will to change, check out the following exercise. Ask yourself how much you really believe:

1) that you actually do have diabetes;

2) that the disease can have serious consequences;

3) that following the advice of your healthcare givers will benefit your health;

4) that the benefits of treatment cancel out the inconveniences;

5) that you feel capable of putting into practice the advice of caregivers.

5. Can myths about the disease and its treatment become obstacles to the will to change?

Certainly. Myths created from false information, rumours, family stories, urban legends and cultural perceptions can all play a negative role. Often, they become justifications used to avoid taking care of yourself, to treat yourself inadequately or to abandon a treatment that you may not understand well.

Common myths among people with diabetes

- If I take pills to treat my diabetes, I can eat whatever I want.
- My diabetes is "minor", in fact my "sugar levels" are just a "ting bit high", and therefore I do not need treatment.
- I have to eliminate all sugars from my diet.
- Taking medications to treat diabetes causes a physical dependence because they are "chemicals", and therefore they should be taken as little as possible.
- If I inject insulin, I will become a "junkie."
- I got diabetes because I ate too much sugar.
- Diabetes treated with insulin is much worse than diabetes treated with oral antidiabetic medications.
- My diabetes is cured because my blood glucose level has returned to normal.
- Since I do not have any obvious symptoms, I must not have the disease.
- If I ignore the problems, they will disappear.
- No matter what I do, I am still going to end up with complications and end up dying, so what is the use?

---

6. What can you do to reinforce the positive effects of your health beliefs and reduce the negative effects of myths on the will to change?

1) Assess your health beliefs on a regular basis.

2) Examine your personal convictions about diabetes and its treatment on a regular basis.

3) Look for information:

➤ read up on diabetes;

➤ speak to your doctor;

➤ take a training course at a diabetes teaching centre;

➤ exchange information on diabetes with others.

7. What are the steps involved in changing your behaviour?

The following chart presents the steps for change. Learning about these steps can help you to identify the actions that will enable you to progress from one step to the next.

Step	Description	Action
Precontemplation	You have no intention of changing your behaviour.	1) Remain open to change. 2) Look for information that can make you more aware of the importance of the changes you must make.
Contemplation	You have started to think about making changes in the coming six months.	1) Identify the obstacles to change. 2) Assess the advantages and disadvantages of change. 3) Ask the people around you for help.
Preparation	You have decided to make a change during the next month.	1) Establish a plan that sets clear goals. 2) Making a verbal agreement with your doctor or spouse can prove to be very useful.
Action	You have made a change. You have maintained it for fewer than six months.	Look for support, especially during periods when you are most vulnerable, such as vacations or periods of exceptional stress.
Maintenance	You have made a change. You have maintained it for at least six months.	Reward yourself if you have achieved your goal (e.g., treat yourself to a massage or set aside some money for a night out).

8.   How can you set attainable and realistic goals for yourself?

Here are the elements that should be taken into account in order to increase the likelihood of reaching your goals. Your goals should be:

1)   specific:

The plan must be clear. For example, instead of saying "I will eat more regularly," it is better to specifically say "I will eat three meals a day, five out of seven days."

2)   measurable:

It is easier to assess your progress when goals can be checked or measured.

3)   self-directed:

You must participate in establishing your goals. They are your goals.

4)   realistic:

Outline small challenges that you are likely to meet. Remember, success breeds success.

5)   defined according to a deadline or time frame:

Set a start date and a time limit, and keep track of your progress.

6)   assessed in terms of the support expected:

Determine whether you need the support of your family, friends or caregivers to help you reach your goal.

9.   What strategies can motivate you to exercise more?

1)   Exercise with a goal in mind:

Walking the dog or biking to work, for example.

2)   Start off slowly:

It is better to walk only 10 minutes a day than not to walk at all.

3) **Remind yourself of the benefits of exercise:**

Exercise is known to be an excellent way to combat stress and depression, and to protect you from heart disease. It also helps control blood glucose levels in people with diabetes.

4) **Make exercise a regular part of your life:**

Program your exercise regimen in the same way you plan your work schedule or your social activities.

5) **Be flexible:**

Engage in the kind of exercise suits you best in terms of schedule, budget and abilities.

6) **Make exercise enjoyable:**

Vary your physical activities to see which ones are the most enjoyable.

7) **Exercise with other people:**

Find partners with whom to walk, play tennis, work out, or with whom to enjoy activities set in nature, like hiking and bird watching.

10. What strategies can motivate you to eat better?

Following a meal plan is probably the most difficult part of diabetes treatment. Here are several suggestions to help you get there.

1) Work out a clear and realistic meal plan with your dietician.

2) Modify your environment to reach your objectives more easily. For example, do not buy cookies if you know you cannot resist them.

3) Keep things in perspective when you seem to fall short of your goals. For example, use glycosylated hemogoblin instead of just the week's blood glucose levels to assess the impact of weight loss on your diabetes control.

4)   Beware of and check your tendency to go to extremes. For example, do not be too strict or deprive yourself of too much at one time, because this can often provoke a reactive desire to overindulge.

5)   Focus your attention on the new, good habits that should to be developed rather than on the bad ones that should be abandoned.

6)   If your day-to-day routine is monotonous, and eating has become the only pleasant and stimulating activity in your life, you must seriously consider reorganizing things. For example, become a volunteer, join an activity club, or take up a hobby.

7)   Build up your self-assertion skills, especially if you are a person who finds it difficult to say no.

---

[1] Taken from the book *Diabetes Burnout: What to Do When You Can't Take It Anymore*, by W. Polonsky. Alexandria, VA; American Diabetes Association, 1999.

CHAPTER 27
Sex and Family Planning

1. Can having diabetes affect a person's sex life?

For women as well as for men, diabetes can cause problems that affect sexual function. However, in women, these problems are more discreet and do not directly impede the sex act; by the same token, there has been less research into sexual dysfunction in women, and hence less is understood about it. In men, on the other hand, we know that chronically elevated blood glucose levels can result in difficulty achieving and maintaining an erection, and thus in the inability to have satisfactory sexual relations: this is called **erectile dysfunction.**

2. Do all men with diabetes suffer from erectile dysfunction?

No. Not all men with diabetes necessarily develop erectile dysfunction.

3. How can diabetes cause erectile dysfunction in men?

Over a period of time, hyperglycemia can cause two problems in penis function:

1) damage to nerves, and

2) thickening and hardening of the arteries, which may compromise circulation.

These two problems, separately or in combination, can result in a partial or complete inability to have an erection (hence erectile dysfunction).

Poorly controlled diabetes can affect the condition of your overall health, which can in turn cause erectile dysfunction. In this case, correcting the hyperglycemia generally brings about a restoration of normal sexual function.

4. Is erectile dysfunction in men with diabetes always caused by the disease?

No. Erectile dysfunction in men with diabetes is often due to factors and causes that have nothing to do with the disease. These include:

1) medication;

2) hormonal problems;

3) psychological problems.

5. How can erectile dysfunction be prevented in men with diabetes?

The following steps can be taken to decrease the risk of erectile dysfunction:

1) keep blood glucose levels as close to normal as possible;

2) follow your meal plan's recommendations concerning fats;

3) quit smoking, if applicable;

4) maintain good control of hypertension and all blood lipid abnormalities;

5) stop or decrease alcohol consumption, if applicable.

6. How is erectile dysfunction assessed?

The following tests are performed to assess erectile dysfunction:

1) Doppler test, which examines penile blood flow;

2) electromyography (EMG) of the penis, in order to measure neurological conductivity;

3) measurements of hormone levels;

4) evaluation of nocturnal erections; the presence of nocturnal erections suggests that the erectile dysfunction is of psychological origin;

5) psychological evaluation if the preceding tests are negative.

7. Can erectile dysfunction in men with diabetes be treated?

Yes. The key is to identify the problem that causes this dysfunction in order to treat it appropriately. The following issues should be explored:

1) in some cases, better control of blood glucose is beneficial;

2) any hormonal problem must be corrected;

3) any medication that inhibits sexual function must be eliminated, if possible;

4) certain medications and treatments may induce an erection and eventually make full sexual relations possible, including:

➡ oral medications such as Viagra®, Cialis® or Levitra®;

➡ insertion of prostaglandin suppositories (Muse®) into the urethra;

➡ injection of prostaglandin at the base of the penis (Caverject®);

5) in the case of severe organic erectile dysfunction, a penile prosthetic device may be used;

6) finally, sexual therapy given by a sexologist often proves beneficial, either by helping the individual adapt to his sexual difficulties or by resolving psychological conflicts at the root of the sexual problem.

8. Are there risks associated with pregnancy in women with diabetes?

Yes. Pregnancy can generate certain risks for diabetic women, especially if blood glucose is poorly controlled. There are three types of risks:

1)   risks to the mother:

- worsening of diabetic complications;
- urinary infections;
- acidosis in women with type 1 diabetes;
- serious hypoglycemia.

2)   risks to the baby:

- spontaneous miscarriage;
- malformations;
- death in utero;
- premature birth;
- hypoglycemia at birth.

3)   risks to both mother and baby:

- toxemia of pregnancy, characterized by hypertension, protein in the urine and edema (fluid overload) in the lower limbs

9. How can pregnancy complications be prevented in women with diabetes?

It is usually possible to prevent these complications. A woman with diabetes **must absolutely see her physician** before deciding to become pregnant. It is very important to:

1)   assess and treat complications that might worsen during pregnancy, especially those involving the eyes;

2)   control blood glucose as effectively as possible to limit any associated risks.

Only when these issues have been addressed should a woman with diabetes consider becoming pregnant.

10. Are there complications related to diabetes that put a woman with the disease at particular risk during pregnancy?

Yes. Certain complications related to diabetes put a pregnant woman at particular risk, especially if her blood glucose is poorly controlled. These include the risks of:

1) progression of retinopathy;

2) progression of kidney damage with severe loss of renal function;

3) serious hypertension;

4) heart failure, if there has been prior cardiac damage.

If these complications develop, the termination of pregnancy for medical reasons may have to be considered.

11. What are the risks that the baby may develop diabetes if one of the parents has the disease?

If one of the parents has **type 1 diabetes**, the risk of the baby developing the disease in the long term is **5%**.

If one of the parents has **type 2 diabetes**, the risk of the baby developing the disease in the long term is **25%**.

12. What contraceptive methods are available to women with diabetes?

There are no contraceptive methods specifically designed for women with diabetes. However, certain contraceptive methods entail greater risks for them. There are two types of methods:

1) **hormonal contraception:**

   ➤ **"combined" pills** containing two hormones – estrogen and progesterone. This form of birth control is effective, but may carry certain risks on blood glucose levels and blood vessels;

➡ **"low-dose progestin"** containing a small amount of progestin. This is an effective method of contraception and it has little effect on blood glucose levels. However, the long-term effects of this form of birth control on the blood vessels are unknown;

➡ intramuscular injections or intra-uterine devices (IUDs) with progestin. These are effective forms of birth control that have no effect on blood glucose or on blood vessels;

2)   mechanical contraception:

➡ intrauterine devices (IUDs) are effective and pose no additional risk of infection, provided the woman with diabetes controls her blood glucose properly;

➡ barrier methods such as condoms, diaphragms and spermicides can be used without risk by women with diabetes. However, these methods are less effective.

The choice of a contraceptive method should be guided by the following considerations: woman's age, the duration of the diabetes and its level of control, the presence of diabetic complications, whether or not the woman is a smoker, the number of previous pregnancies, the effectiveness of the method and, of course, the preferences of the woman and her partner.

13. Can a woman with diabetes safely use emergency oral contraception?

Emergency oral contraceptives, otherwise known as postcoital contraception or "the morning after pill," are not contraindicated for women with diabetes. This contraceptive method can be used after unprotected sexual relations. However, it is not recommended for regular contraceptive usage. It involves taking an oral contraceptive according to one of the following methods:

1)   a 100 mg dose of ethinylestradiol (an estrogen) combined with 500 mg of levonorgestrel (a progestin) as soon as possible after sexual relations, and a second dose 12 hours later (e.g., two doses of two Ovral® tablets); or

2) a 750 mg dose of levonorgestrel (Plan B®) as soon as possible after sexual relations and a second dose 12 hours later.

Emergency oral contraceptives must be prescribed by a doctor or, in the province of Quebec, by a doctor or a pharmacist.

14. What methods of sterilization are available?

Sterilization is an option that should be considered by women who have had a number of pregnancies, especially if diabetes-related complications have developed. The options are:

1) for women, tubal ligation

2) for men, vasectomy

15. Can a menopausal woman with diabetes take hormones?

A menopausal woman with diabetes can take hormones, namely, estrogens with or without progestins.

However, it has recently been shown that combined hormonal therapy (estrogens and progestins) in menopausal women can be associated with a minimal but significant risk of breast cancer, thrombophlebitis (blood clots), stroke and coronary disease. Therefore, menopausal women should only be treated with hormones (estrogens and progestins) if the menopausal symptoms cause major discomfort (e.g., hot flashes), and only for a maximum of four years. Afterwards, medication should be discontinued if the symptoms have disappeared.

The following should be considered when deciding whether to take estrogens:

1) prior thrombophlebitis;

2) prior cerebrovascular problems, especially in women who smoke;

3) prior history of breast cancer in the family.

CHAPTER 28

Research: Outlook for the Future

Thanks to some exciting breakthroughs and continued progress in research, we have entered the third millennium with a better understanding of the causes of diabetes and its complications, thus offering increased hope for people with the condition.

In type 1 diabetes, it appears that a change in the insulin-producing cells of the pancreas, caused by environmental factors (such as viral infections), prevents the body from recognizing its own cells and prompts it to make antibodies to destroy these cells. This ability of the body to make antibodies against its own cells seems to be genetically transmitted. The good news is that we have discovered that these antibodies can be detected about five years before the appearance of the disease.

In type 2 diabetes, two major factors intervene in the development of the disease: resistance to insulin (which results in much more insulin being needed to maintain normal blood glucose levels) and a decrease in the capacity of pancreatic cells to produce insulin. In most cases, insulin resistance occurs several years before the development of diabetes. As long as the pancreatic cells can compensate by producing more insulin, blood glucose levels remain normal. Only when pancreatic cells can no longer compensate and insulin production decreases do blood glucose levels rise. The first sign we see is the increase of blood glucose levels, especially after meals, which is called impaired glucose tolerance – this is the pre-diabetic stage. If insulin production decreases further, blood glucose levels will rise even higher after meals and, finally, even before meals – this is when diabetes appears. Susceptibility to insulin resistance and the decreased capacity to produce insulin are partly genetically transmitted. Moreover, we now know that excess weight and physical inactivity will increase resistance to insulin and thus, in genetically susceptible people, increase the risk of developing diabetes.

Over the last decade, two major studies have definitively confirmed that complications due to diabetes are principally related to high blood glucose levels over the course of several years. The first study, a Canadian-American trial (DCCT) published in 1993, followed 1,440 patients with type 1 diabetes. The second, a British trial (UKPDS) published in 1998, followed over 5,000 patients with type 2 diabetes. The two studies concluded that diabetes, whether of type 1 or type 2, must be treated aggressively to maintain blood glucose levels as close to normal as possible in order to prevent complications related to the disease.

Clearly, this is a great challenge. However, thanks to significant strides made in diabetes research, we can count on new pharmacological and technological developments that will help us not only to improve the control of blood glucose, but perhaps also to cure and even prevent the disease and its complications.

The DCCT and UKPDS studies also demonstrated the difficulty in achieving a normal blood glucose level. Getting there will require new medications. Several **antidiabetic drugs** are currently being studied, such as:

1) drugs that delay the absorption of sugar in the intestine (e.g., GLP-analogue, excendin-4 and pramlintide);

2) drugs that stimulate the secretion of insulin by the pancreas (e.g., GLP-1 analogue, excendin-4 and pramlintide);

3) long-acting insulin analogues (e.g., glargine insulin and detemir insulin) and rapid-acting insulin analogues (e.g., glulisine);

4) new ways to administer insulin – inhalable insulin (e.g., Exubera®) absorbed by the lungs, and oral insulin (e.g., Oralin®) absorbed by the buccal mucosa.

Pancreas transplants have already been successfully performed in many Canadian hospitals. The two major problems we have encountered, however, are the shortage of donors and the side effects of anti-rejection drugs. Nevertheless, progress has recently been made in **islets of Langerhans transplantation**, a procedure that consists of injecting the pancreatic cells (whose job it is to manufacture insulin). A group of

Canadian researchers in Edmonton showed innovation in improving the technique (referred to as the "Edmonton Protocol") of isolating islets and by using new combinations of anti-rejection drugs (without cortisone). In the Edmonton Protocol technique, ambulatory transplants are performed under local anaesthesia. A catheter is inserted into the portal vein entering the liver, and the islets are injected, using a syringe. Up until this point, several dozen patients have undergone the transplant successfully, and the long-term benefits are encouraging. One difficulty, though, is that the isolation technique only allows for the recovery of 20% of the islets, requiring two and sometimes three transplantations of islets before blood glucose can be normalized. The problem of donor shortage is therefore made all the more acute. However, improved techniques for isolating islets should partially solve this problem.

New avenues are also being explored with a view to finding insulin-producing and secreting cells for transplant. **Genetic engineering** allows us to take intestine cells, for example, and then genetically program them to make insulin. Here is the way this works. In the intestine, there are specialized cells that secrete a hormone called GLP-1, which is controlled by glucose. These cells respond to changes in blood glucose: The increase in blood glucose stimulates an increase in the production and secretion of the hormone, and the decrease of blood glucose in turn then decreases the production and secretion of the hormone. If we genetically reprogram the cells to make insulin, they will be stimulated by hyperglycemia, and their numbers will be curbed by the lowering of blood glucose levels. Researchers have demonstrated that this is possible in mice, and can cure diabetes at the animal level – without the need for anti-rejection drugs. Before we move from mice to humans, there remains a lot of work to do, but this dream is within the realm of the possible!

Over the past few years, much has been discussed about embryo stem cells or, more recently, about stem cells from adult human bone marrow. These stem cells can transform themselves into any mature cell, including pancreatic cells capable of producing insulin. These first steps are very encouraging.

The **prevention of complications** due to diabetes remains a major challenge for researchers. Thanks to a greater understanding of the physiopathological mechanisms responsible for these complications, several studies are currently evaluating new drugs that could prevent complications due to diabetes, independent of the control of blood glucose. We have already emphasized the importance of high blood glucose levels in the development of diabetic complications. Several studies have demonstrated that high blood glucose levels are associated with overproduction of an enzyme known as protein kinase C, and have shown that it is involved in the development of complications. The pharmaceutical industry has perfected an inhibitor of protein kinase C and shown that this drug can prevent complications in diabetic animals. Studies in humans are currently underway. Such a drug may eventually prevent the development of complications, despite the difficulty in achieving optimal control of blood glucose.

The ultimate goal of research remains the **prevention of diabetes**.

We know that in type 1 diabetes, the pancreatic cells that produce insulin are destroyed by antibodies. We can measure the appearance of these antibodies about five years before the disease develops in people at risk. Some studies in this high-risk group have investigated the possibility of preventing the disease through treatments that block the production of antibodies as soon as they appear. Thus far, these studies have come up negative. The only ongoing study on preventing type 1 diabetes is an international nutritional one. Clearly, we need to better understand the cause of type 1 diabetes before we can prevent the disease. Numerous studies in this domain are currently underway in Canada and at the international level.

We know that in type 2 diabetes, the disease is preceded by a "pre-diabetic" phase called "impaired glucose tolerance." The impaired glucose tolerance phase can be easily identified. A Finnish study and an American one have recently shown that a weight reducing diet and exercise can reduce the risk of type 2 diabetes by as much as 58% in subjects with impaired glucose tolerance. The American study also demonstrated that metformin can decrease the risk of diabetes by 31% in subjects with impaired glucose intolerance. More recently, a Canadian study (STOP-NIDDM) showed that acarbose can decrease the risk of diabetes by 36% in subjects in the pre-diabetic stage. Other studies on prevention are currently underway, including the DREAM study, which is looking into the effect of ramipril and rosiglitazone on the prevention of type 2 diabetes.

All of these research projects are being carried out at the international level, with the active participation of many Canadian researchers. Each one brings hope to people with diabetes.

CHAPTER 29

Tools for Following Up on Diabetes

1. How can you "manage" your diabetes?

Managing diabetes involves a number of challenges. Medical follow-ups, self-monitoring of blood glucose, diet, exercise and medication are all important aspects of treatment for a person with diabetes.

These responsibilities may seem overwhelming, all the more so since diabetes makes you reconsider your entire lifestyle, and requires a long-term commitment on your part in order to manage the condition properly. To improve your treatment, therefore, you may want to take things one step at a time rather than trying to change all your habits at once. Set clear and realistic goals, **congratulate yourself for each goal reached successfully and all difficulties overcome.**

2. Are there tools that can help you follow up on your diabetes?

A person with diabetes can rely on several tools that will help in the follow-up of the disease. Your self-monitoring logbook is obviously essential. A "journal of personal goals" is another useful tool. It should list the goals relevant to a person with diabetes, particularly those related to five important aspects of the follow-up: medical follow-up, care, diet, medication and wellbeing. You should choose one to five goals, among all those listed, that you deem the most important. You can then number them in terms of priority (e.g., 1 to 5).

It is advisable to consult your "journal of personal goals" from time to time. Checking it periodically can help you to keep track of progress, to understand why some goals are difficult to reach, to determine the means required to reach them or to set new objectives. See the example offered at the end of this chapter for more details.

3.   Is there a tool to help manage the dietary aspect of diabetes?

A meal plan is a very useful tool for a person with diabetes. It is drawn up with the help of your dietician.

4.   Which tests and targets help achieve optimal control of diabetes?

The medical follow-up of a person with diabetes includes various tests: blood glucose, glycosylated hemoglobin (A1C), lipid profile and blood pressure.

Target values for the various tests or measurements are presented in the "Targets for optimal control" chart.

5.   What is the value of test results?

Test results allow a doctor to choose the appropriate treatment for a person with diabetes, and then to assess its effectiveness and adjust it accordingly. The "Test follow-up journal" can be used to keep track of relevant information, including test results. These results allow a person with diabetes to follow treatment as it evolves, discuss it with his or her doctor, and may also serve as a motivational tool.

JOURNAL OF PERSONAL GOALS

Here is a list of relevant goals for a person with diabetes. Choose those that are the most important to you (a maximum of 5) and prioritize them. Revise these objectives periodically.

DATE					
MEDICAL FOLLOW-UP					
See my doctor at least twice a year					
Inquire about the results of analyses and tests performed					
Check my blood pressure regularly					
Check my microalbuminuria once a year					
See my ophthalmologist regularly, as recommended					
CARE AND RECOMMENDATIONS					
Write down my blood glucose levels in my self-monitoring logbook, and analyze them as recommended					
In case of illness, check my blood glucose level more often					
Compare readings from my glucose meter with a blood test at least once a year					
Carry carbohydrates with me at all times (at least two portions of 15-g each)					
Examine my feet every day					
Do not smoke					
Exercise regularly (every day, if possible)					
Wear a bracelet or pendant identifying me as a person with diabetes					

Concerning your driving licence, inform authorities about your condition					
DIET					
Eat the recommended amount of carbohydrates for each meal					
Eat balanced meals (carbohydrates, proteins, fats)					
Choose fibre-rich foods					
Eat snacks in the evening, as recommended					
Keep regular mealtimes					
Measure my food portions from time to time					
Keep a regular food journal					
Eat the fats recommended by my health care team					
Only drink alcohol when I eat					
MEDICATION					
Take medications as prescribed by my doctor					
Know the names of my antidiabetic medications					
Write down all the antidiabetic medications I take and any changes of dosage in my self-monitoring logbook					
Keep a completely up-to-date list of all my medications (names, doses) and bring it to medical appointments					
Follow the adjustment rules for insulin doses					
Know the best times to take my medications					
Know how to deal with any skipped doses of my antidiabetic medications					
Make sure that over-the-counter medications or natural products that I take do not worsen my condition					

WELL-BEING					
Identify the stress factors that affect me most					
Improve my reactions to stress					
Set aside at least 10 minutes a day for relaxation					
Speak to my support network about my diabetes					
Manage my time in a way that matches my needs					
MY PERSONAL GOALS					

Signature : _____

TARGETS FOR OPTIMAL CONTROL

Glucose	
Glycosylated hemoglobin (A1C)	≤ 0.070 (≤ 0.060, if possible)
Fasting blood glucose or before meals	4 mmol/l–7 mmol/l (4 mmol/l–6 mmol/l, if possible)
Blood glucose 1 to 2 hours after meals	5 mmol/l–10 mmol/l (5 mmol/l–8 mmol/l, if possible)
Lipid profile	
LDL cholesterol	< 2.5 mmol/l
Total cholesterol/HDL-cholesterol	< 4
Triglycerides	< 1.5 mmol/l
Kidneys	
Albumin/creatinine ratio	M: < 2.0 mg/mmoL; F: < 2.8 mg/mmol
Microalbuminuria	< 20 µg/min. or < 30 mg/day
Other	
Blood pressure	≤ 130/80 mmHg
Normal weight	< 65 years: BMI* 18.5–24.9 ≥ 65 years: BMI 18.6–29.9
Waist	M: < 102 cm; F: < 88 cm

* BMI: body mass index (weight in kg/height in m^2)

Name: _____

TEST FOLLOW-UP JOURNAL

Date							
Weight (kg)							
Height (m)							
BMI (kg/m^2)							
Waist (cm)							
Blood pressure (≤ 130/80 mmHg)							
Blood glucose (blood test): Before meals: 4 mmol/l–7 mmol/l (4 mmol/l–6 mmol/l, if possible) After meals: 5 mmol/l–10 mmol/l (5 mmol/l–8 mmol/l, if possible)							
Glycosylated hemoglobin (A1C) (≤ 0.070 or ≤ 0.060, if possible)							
Triglycerides (< 1.5 mmol/l)							
LDL-cholesterol (< 2.5 mmol/l)							
HDL-cholesterol (>1.0 mmol/l)							
Total cholesterol / HDL-cholesterol (< 4)							
Albumin/creatinine ratio (M: < 2.0 mg/mmol; F: < 2.8 mg/mmol)							
Microalbuminuria (< 20 µg/min. or < 30 mg/day)							
Creatinine clearance (1.2 ml/s–2.4 ml/s)							

BLOOD GLUCOSE CONVERSION CHART

mmol/l*	mg/dL**	mmol/l	mg/dL
1.4	25	11.2	202
1.6	29	11.6	209
1.8	32	12.0	216
2.0	36	12.4	223
2.4	43	12.8	230
2.8	50	13.2	238
3.2	58	13.6	245
3.6	65	14.0	252
4.0	72	14.4	259
4.4	79	14.8	266
4.8	86	15.2	274
5.2	94	15.6	281
5.6	101	16.0	288
6.0	108	16.4	295
6.4	115	16.8	302
6.8	122	17.2	309
7.0	126	17.6	317
7.2	130	18.0	324
7.6	137	18.5	333
8.0	144	19.0	342
8.4	151	19.5	351
8.8	158	20.0	360
9.2	166	20.5	369
9.6	173	21.0	378
10.0	180	21.5	387
10.4	187	22.0	396
10.8	194	22.5	405

Target values before meals and at bedtime (shaded region: 4.0 to 7.0 mmol/l, 72 to 126 mg/dL)

* mmol/l x 18 = mg/dL

** mg/dL ÷ 18 = mmol/l

Annexe II

Community Resources

Some publications written for people with diabetes

➤   Diabetes Dialogue
Published by :
Canadian Diabetes Association
522 University Avenue, 13th floor
Toronto (Ontario) M5G 1Y7
☎ (416) 363-3373
🖰 Website: www.diabetes.ca

➤   Plein soleil
Published by :
Diabetes Québec
8550 Pie-IX Blvd., suite 300
Montreal (Quebec) H1Z 4G2
☎ (514) 259-3422 or (toll free) 1 800 361-3504
🖰 Website: www.diabete.qc.ca
🖰 Email: info@diabete.qc.ca

➤   Diabetes Forecast
Published by:
American Diabetes Association
1701 North Beauregard Street
Alexandria, VA 22311

UNITED STATES

☎ Toll-free: 1 800 342-2383
🖱 Website: www.diabetes.org

Websites dealing with diabetes

➤ American Diabetes Association
🖱 www.diabetes.org

➤ American Dietetic Association
🖱 www.webdietitians.org

➤ Canadian Diabetes Association
🖱 www.diabetes.ca

➤ CDC Diabetes Public Health Resource
🖱 www.cdc.gov/diabetes

➤ Children with Diabetes
🖱 www.childrenwithdiabetes.com/index_cwd.htm

➤ Diabetes Québec
🖱 www.diabete.qc.ca

➤ Diabetes Insight
🖱 www.diabetic.org.uk

➤ Diabetes.com Health Library
🖱 www.diabetes.com/tools/health_library/index.html

➤ European Association for the Study of Diabetes
🖱 www.easd.org

➤ International Diabetes Federation
🖱 www.idf.org

➤ Joslin Diabetes Center
🖱 www.joslin.harvard.edu

➤ Juvenile Diabetes Research Foundation Canada
🖱 www.jdfc.ca

➤ Medline plus: diabetes
🖱 www.nlm.nih.gov/medlineplus/diabetes.html

➤ National Diabetes Education Program
🖱 www.ndep.nih.gov

➤ National Institute of Diabetes & Digestive & Kidney Diseases
🖱 www.niddk.nih.gov/health/diabetes/diabetes.htm

➤ National Institutes of Health
🖱 www.niddk.nih.gov

➤ Pancreatic islets transplantation
🖱 http://islet.com